Review Questions for
PHYSICIAN ASSISTANT CERTIFYING EXAMINATIONS

Review Questions for
PHYSICIAN ASSISTANT CERTIFYING EXAMINATIONS

David F. Irvine, MS, RPA-C

Associate Director, Albany-Hudson Valley Physician Assistant Program
Albany Medical College, Albany, New York

Review Questions Series
Series Editor: Thomas R. Gest, PhD
University of Arkansas for Medical Sciences

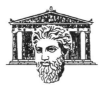

The Parthenon Publishing Group Inc.
International Publishers in Medicine, Science & Technology

One Blue Hill Plaza, Pearl River, New York 10965, USA

Published in the USA by
The Parthenon Publishing Group Inc.
One Blue Hill Plaza,
PO Box 1564, Pearl River,
New York 10965, USA

Published in the UK and Europe by
The Parthenon Publishing Group Limited
Casterton Hall, Carnforth,
Lancs LA6 2LA, UK

Library of Congress Cataloging-in-Publication Data

Irvine, David, REMT-I.
    Review questions for physician assistant certifying examinations / by
David F. Irvine
        p.   cm. -- (Review questions series)
    Includes bibliographic references.
    ISBN: 1-85070-663-8
    1. Physicians' assistants -- Examinations, questions, etc.
    2. Physicians' assistants -- Education. I. Title. II. Title: Physician assistant
examination. III. Series.
    [DNLM: 1. Physician Assistants examination questions. W 18.2 I72r 1998]
R697.P45I78   1998
610.69'53 -- DC21
DNLM/DLC
for Library of Congress   98-14472
                                                                                    CIP

British Library Cataloguing in Publication Data

Irvine, David
    Review questions for physician assistant certifying examinations. – (Review
questions series)
    1. Physicians' assistants – Examinations, questions, etc.
    I. Title
    610.6'953'076

    ISBN 1-85070-663-8

This edition published 1998

Printed in the USA

INTRODUCTION

This book is designed to help prepare the user for the physician assistant certifying examinations administered by the National Commission on the Certification of Physician Assistants (NCCPA). It is intended for individuals sitting for either their initial certification or a subsequent recertification. It is based on the objectives, practice settings, and disease lists identified by the NCCPA for use in developing the certifying exams.

An overall test plan identifying the systems and tasks assessed by the questions in this volume appears following this introduction. With this information, you can compute subscores for individual systems (e.g., nervous system = number correct/50). By working through the individual tests, you can prepare for the exam and calculate subscores by specialty area. These scores can be used to diagnose areas of weakness and direct you to additional preparation.

Each chapter also contains its own test plan at the end of the chapter. These plans, based on the list published by the NCCPA, specify the diseases, disorders, or conditions encompassed by the area, as well as those contained in the chapter, together with the PA tasks being assessed. You can use these plans to identify specific areas of weakness (disease or condition) or specific tasks with which you may have difficulty (e.g., diagnostic studies). This may lead you to use a different type of resource to help you prepare for the exams.

Questions in this book are exclusively type "A" multiple choice, as the NCCPA has eliminated the "K" format from the initial certifying exam and is phasing it out of the recertifying exam. The questions are based on a bibliography of texts used in the instruction of PA students.

Additional emphasis has been placed on physical assessment, as the NCCPA has eliminated the clinical skills component of the exam in favor of all-written testing and will be adding questions in this area.

Some Tips on Preparing for the Certifying Exam

The goal of the NCCPA exam is to assess minimum competence to practice as a PA. The goal of PA education is to prepare at least minimally competent PAs. Therefore, the entire process of PA education (and continuing medical education) is, and should be, an integral part of preparing for the exam. Board preparation should be an ongoing process that begins with enrollment in a PA program—not something to do in a 1-week seminar just prior to the exam.

Test-taking is a learned skill, and you can improve your scores if you work at becoming a better test-taker. Most schools will have a learning assistance center that will provide instruction in test-taking. You should utilize this resource, even if your skills are already good, as even a small improvement may make a difference in your scores.

Recertifying PAs can access this type of instruction at almost any local community college. Also, numerous references (e.g., Vitale B, Nugent P. *Test Success: Test-Taking Techniques for the Health Care Student*. Philadelphia: FA Davis, 1996) also provide specifics on test-taking strategy.

Practice, practice, practice. You should get as many different review questions as you can, use the relevant sections to prepare for rotations, and review for rotation exams throughout your clinical year.

The more you test, the better you will perform. PAs in practice should continue to take CME tests as they follow the journals, as this is the easiest way to keep current, log mandatory CME credits, and prepare for recertification. Don't limit your readings to areas of interest or practice. Identify areas that you do not commonly see in practice and consider CMEs and/or readings to refresh those areas prior to the exam. Personally, I have found the national conference to be very helpful for this purpose. Remember to read all topics listed on the test plan. Use review books diagnostically to identify areas of weakness.

Do not write in your review books. You can go back to those same questions several times for reinforcement before you "know the question." The first time you use a set of questions, practice under "board-like" conditions, allowing 45 seconds per question in the test. Record your answers, and grade yourself before you review the discussion paragraphs. Use this information to direct your studies to areas of weakness during your rotations or in selecting CME sessions. Retake the questions at least one more time in preparation for the end of rotation exam or after reading or attending a CME session.

Remember that a PA career is a commitment to lifelong learning and the "boards" are nothing more or less than a verification of your achieving that commitment.

David F. Irvine
Albany, New York

OVERALL TEST PLAN FOR REVIEW QUESTIONS

Section	1 CNS	2 EYE	3 ENT	4 RESP	5 CV	6 GI	7 PSY	8 MS	9 DERM	10 ENDO NUTR MET	11 REN URO	12 REPR	13 OB NEO	14 HEME	15 ID	16 INJ WNDS BURNS	17 ILL-DEF S/S	Total	%*
Total questions	50	30	60	60	91	65	30	75	45	30	44	45	25	30	61	29	30	800	100
%*	6	4	8	8	11	8	4	9	6	4	5	6	3	4	8	4	4	100	
Tasks/areas assessed																			
Hx and PE	14	1	2	13	17	29	4	30	13	8	11	14	6	5	2	0	6	175	22
Dx studies	2	5	7	9	23	4	0	10	2	5	11	2	1	5	9	2	2	99	12
Diagnosis	10	5	16	8	10	3	6	3	8	3	3	10	1	4	10	5	7	112	14
Prognosis	2	0	1	4	3	4	0	0	5	0	1	0	2	0	2	1	2	27	3
Management																			
Health maintenance	1	0	2	6	5	3	1	2	2	3	4	4	2	3	12	1	0	51	6
Clinical intervention	2	3	4	6	6	3	3	3	2	2	1	0	2	3	3	9	3	55	7
Clinical therapeutics	1	6	11	8	4	5	5	4	3	4	1	3	2	2	11	4	1	75	9
Applying scientific concepts	18	10	17	6	23	14	11	23	10	5	12	12	9	8	12	7	9	206	26

* Individual percentages are rounded to the nearest whole number.

CONTENTS

Introduction vii

✓ 1   Nerv...1

✓ 2   Eye...11

✓ 3   Ear, ...18

✓ 4   Respi..31

✓ 5   Circul...42

✓ 6   Digest...59

✓ 7   Emotic...71

✓ 8   Muscu...77

✓ 9   Skin an...92

✓ 10   Endocri...100

✓ 11   Kidneys...107

✓ 12   Male an..ns.............................115

✓ 13   Pregnan...123

✓ 14   Blood an...128

✓ 15   Infectious Diseases 135

16   Injuries, Wounds, Toxic Effects, and Burns.........................146

17   Ill-Defined Symptom Complexes.......................................152

Bibliography 159

Bookstore re: Grad

$47.50/

25 ø/ return open return of going but

lwk bef grad pick-up

— Call c̄ head size in inches

4/13/49

7 1/8"

1-800-777-3921

SECTION 1: NERVOUS SYSTEM

1.001 A 37-year-old woman comes to you with a 5-day history of severe, right-sided facial pain that is brought on by eating. She describes the pain as "knife-like" and so severe that she has not eaten solid food in 3 days. She has never suffered this in the past. She denies visual changes, tearing, or nasal congestion. Neuro exam is normal. The MOST likely diagnosis is:
   A. cluster headache
   B. migraine headache
   C. subarachnoid hemorrhage
   D. trigeminal neuralgia

D is correct.
This presentation is classic for trigeminal neuralgia, especially the characteristics of the pain. A subarachnoid hemorrhage might be expected to result in neurological deficits; a new onset of migraine is much less likely at this age and typically results in unilateral throbbing pain with or without an aura. Cluster headaches are more common in middle-aged males and are often associated with lacrimation and nasal congestion.

1.002 A patient exhibits loss of pain and temperature sensation in the dermatomes on the left side from the umbilicus down as a result of a partial spinal cord injury that severed one-half of the cord laterally to the midline. Predict the effect on position and vibratory sense.
   A. no effect
   B. loss of position sense and vibratory sense on left in same dermatomes
   C. loss of position sense and intact vibratory sense on left in same dermatomes
   D. intact position sense and loss of vibratory sense on left in same dermatomes
   E. loss of position sense and vibratory sense on right in same dermatomes

E is correct.
Loss of position and vibration will be distal to the injury on the same side, while pain and temperature sensation will be affected distal to the injury on the opposite side. So the injury here is on the right.

1.003 Counting by serial sevens is usually done:
   A. 7, 14, 21, 28, 35, 42 ...
   B. 100, 93, 86, 79, 72 ...
   C. 7, 49, 343 ...
   D. 1, 8, 15 ...
   E. 49, 42, 35 ...

B is correct.
Reproducibility of results dictates that the exam is done the same way each time.

1.004 A healthy 24-year-old PA student slumps gracefully to the floor without injury during a lab practical. Skin color and vital signs are normal. She denies any premonitory symptoms. The MOST likely cause is:
   A. vasodepressor syncope
   B. micturition syncope
   C. hypoglycemia
   D. hysterical fainting
   E. aortic stenosis

D is correct.
Vasodepressor syncope characteristically causes premonitory symptoms, bradycardia and hypotension. Micturition syncope is associated with emptying a full bladder. Hypoglycemia rarely causes loss of consciousness and is symptomatic. Severe aortic stenosis causes syncope but is usually effort related and is unlikely in this age group.

1.005 A 28-year-old PA student complains of lightheadedness and palpitations on standing up. She states she has been feeling "terrible" for 2 days with frequent bouts of watery diarrhea, vomiting, fever, and chills. She has been unable to keep anything down for 12 hours. This is MOST likely:
  A. massive pulmonary embolism
  B. inadequate vasoconstrictor reflexes
  C. hypovolemia
  D. hysterical fainting
  E. hypertrophic cardiomyopathy

C is correct.
Increased losses in diarrhea, vomiting, and fever combined with inadequate intake make dehydration likely in this person.

1.006 The reason for having a patient focus on a distant object during the funduscopic exam is that it:
  A. keeps eyes still and dilates pupils
  B. keeps eyes still and elicits rotatory nystagmus
  C. dilates pupils and elicits rotatory nystagmus
  D. dilates pupils
  E. keeps eyes still

A is correct.
This keeps the eyes still, but also focusing in the distance dilates the pupils.

1.007 Major risk factors for stroke include:
  A. hypertension
  B. diabetes
  C. smoking
  D. hyperlipidemia
  E. all of the above

E is correct.
Marked similarities occur with cardiovascular risk factors, as atherosclerotic disease is felt to be a contributor to the pathogenesis of strokes.

1.008 A man with a history of untreatable prostate cancer presents to the ER, complaining of sudden onset of severe back pain and bilateral leg weakness. The MOST likely diagnosis is:
  A. herniated disc
  B. muscular back sprain
  C. spondylolysis
  D. compression fracture

D is correct.
Compression fracture with cord compression is likely in a patient with potentially metastatic disease.

1.009 All of the following are components of a reflex arc EXCEPT:
  A. intact sensory nerve fibers
  B. functional synapses in medulla
  C. intact motor nerve fibers
  D. functional neuromuscular junctions
  E. competent muscle fibers

B is correct.
Reflex arcs are limited to the cord at the level of innervation.

1.010 Children with first febrile seizures should receive _____ prophylaxis.
  A. phenobarbital
  B. phenytoin
  C. valproic acid
  D. diazepam
  E. no

E is correct.
Prophylactic treatment for single febrile seizures is not routinely indicated.

1.011 Nystagmus may be caused by:
   A. vision problems in early life
   B. disorders of the labyrinth
   C. cerebellar disease
   D. drug toxicity
   E. all of the above

E is correct.
Similar to tremors in other parts of the body, the causes are multiple.

1.012 Atrial fibrillation is associated with:
   A. ischemic stroke
   B. internal cerebral hemorrhage
   C. epidural hemorrhage
   D. embolic stroke
   E. subdural hemorrhage

D is correct.
Mural thrombi form that are then prone to embolize.

1.013 Pronator drift suggests:
   A. proprioception deficit
   B. sensory deficit
   C. cerebellar dysfunction
   D. early muscle weakness
   E. vestibular dysfunction

D is correct.
Although commonly tested with the Romberg test.

1.014 Three types of tremors include:
   A. static, dyskinesia, intention
   B. resting, postural, intention
   C. static, dystonia, dyskinesia
   D. resting, postural, chorea
   E. resting, dyskinesia, intention

B is correct.
Resting tremors disappear with movement (Parkinson's), intention appear with activity (MS), and postural occur when a certain position is maintained (hyperthyroid).

1.015 Staring is a manifestation of a:
   A. complex partial seizure
   B. myoclonic seizure
   C. absence seizure
   D. tonic-clonic seizure

C is correct.
Also referred to as "petit mal."

1.016 Proper classification of seizure type is important for:
   A. comparison of data regarding drug therapy
   B. appropriate choice of anticonvulsant drug
   C. prognosis
   D. decisions regarding driving
   E. all of the above

E is correct.
Major differences in therapy and prognosis exist among the types of seizures.

1.017 A 52-year-old physician taking Coumadin® for a DVT slips on the cellar stairs, bumping his head and elbow. He sustains no obvious injury at the time. Three weeks later, he complains of mild headache, and his wife notes changes in his personality. The MOST likely diagnosis is:
   A. paranoid psychosis
   B. stroke
   C. chronic subdural hematoma
   D. allergy to Coumadin®
   E. migraine

C is correct.
Anticoagulant therapy puts this patient at risk for bleeding even with minor trauma.

1.018 A known alcoholic is brought to the emergency room, having fallen down a flight of stairs 4 hours earlier. He is stuporous, smells of alcohol, has a bruise on his right temple, and, on painful stimulation, moves his left side poorly. The diagnosis you must rule out first is:

    A. acute subdural hematoma
    B. alcohol intoxication and old stroke
    C. meningitis
    D. brain tumor
    E. alcohol withdrawal seizure

A is correct.
Right-sided trauma with a left-sided motor deficit in an at-risk patient is highly suspicious for subdural.

1.019 The first diagnostic test (of those listed) for the patient in 1.018 is:
    A. CBC
    B. LP
    C. CT scan
    D. LFTs
    E. skull x-rays

C is correct.
CT scan is needed to rule out the subdural.

1.020 A 24-year-old PA student lumps over in his chair during lecture. His classmates state he was up late studying and did not eat anything all day. He appears pale, and on return of consciousness (promptly after lying on floor), he complains of nausea and weakness. He states "you have to do something about the broken air conditioner." The MOST likely diagnosis is:
    A. vasodepressor syncope
    B. micturition syncope
    C. arrhythmia
    D. hysterical fainting
    E. aortic stenosis

A is correct.
Vasovagal episodes account for the majority of this type of syncopal event.

1.021 A 70-year-old man reports sudden loss of consciousness at 3 AM today, while standing to void. He states loss of consciousness was brief with prompt return to normal. He has no past medical history or medications to report. His PE is normal for age. The MOST likely cause is:
    A. vasodepressor syncope
    B. micturition syncope
    C. hypoglycemia
    D. hysterical fainting
    E. aortic stenosis

B is correct.
Associated with emptying a full bladder.

1.022 Hemiparesis can be caused by:
    A. tumor
    B. subdural hematoma
    C. epidural hematoma
    D. stroke
    E. all of the above

E is correct.
Focal motor deficits may be associated with a variety of intracranial events.

1.023 Brain tumors can be treated with all of the following modalities EXCEPT:
   A. radiation therapy
   B. corticosteroid (Decadron®)
   C. mannitol
   D. anticonvulsants (Dilantin®, phenobarbital)
   E. anticoagulants (heparin, warfarin)

E is correct.
Radiation to shrink the tumor, steroids and mannitol for edema, and anticonvulsants to prevent seizures.

1.024 In testing of CN____, the uvula deviates _____ deficit.
   A. IX, away from
   B. X, away from
   C. X, toward
   D. IX, toward
   E. XI, toward

B is correct.
With lesions of the vagal nerve, there is no rise to the palate with "ah" (bilateral), or if unilateral, the palate is pulled away from the affected side.

1.025 When assessing the corneal reflex, you are looking for the normal response of:
   A. blinking on stimulated side only
   B. blinking on stimulated side and constriction of contralateral pupil
   C. blinking on both sides
   D. constriction of ipsilateral pupil and blinking on stimulated side
   E. constriction of both pupils

C is correct.
Sensory CN V and motor CN VII.

1.026 Touch sensation may be preserved despite cord damage because:
   A. the fibers travel in a small, well localized part of the cord
   B. the part of the cord where they travel is well protected
   C. redundant fibers travel via the cranial nerves
   D. fibers travel on both sides of the cord
   E. secondary cutaneous nerves carry impulses around a cord lesion

D is correct.

1.027 Characteristics of a generalized tonic-clonic (grand mal) seizure include:
   A. unimpaired consciousness, blank stare, and automatisms
   B. loss of consciousness, falling, rigid posture, urinary incontinence, and postictal confusion
   C. abnormal stereotyped sensation involving a specific body part.
   D. impaired consciousness without loss of consciousness, lip smacking followed by amnesia for the event
   E. lapse of attention lasting 10–15 seconds without convulsion

B is correct.
Major motor seizures cause loss of consciousness.

1.028 The first step in the management of a patient in status epilepticus is:
    A. insure that the patient has an adequate airway and is breathing well
    B. give IV diazepam
    C. obtain a neuro consult
    D. obtain a head CT
    E. give intravenous phenytoin (Dilantin®)

A is correct.
ABCs first, then the drugs.

1.029 In the testing of a deep tendon reflex, the response is very brisk and clonus is present. What grade would you assign?
    A. 1/4
    B. 2/4
    C. 3/4
    D. 4/4

D is correct.
This is hyperreflexia and suggests upper motor neuron disease.

1.030 A patient presents complaining that her hands shake. On further questioning, you find that the tremor is worse when she tries to do something, especially her cross-stitching. This type of tremor suggests:
    A. fatigue
    B. anxiety
    C. cerebellar disorder
    D. hyperthyroid
    E. familial trait

C is correct.
The others are causes of postural tremors.

1.031 Which of the following sensory perceptions travels in the lateral spinothalamic tract with pain perception?
    A. position sense
    B. vibratory sense
    C. fine touch
    D. temperature

D is correct.
Position, vibration, and fine touch travel in the posterior column

1.032 Following a MVA, the patient is numb from the umbilicus down and is unable to more his legs, though he can move his arms. Transection of the cord occurred at approximately:
    A. T6
    B. T10
    C. T12
    D. L2
    E. L5

B is correct.
The umbilicus is at sensory dermatome T10.

1.033 While assessing a patient, you note two beats of nystagmus in the extreme lateral gaze; this:
    A. suggests a brain stem lesion
    B. suggests a motor cortex lesion
    C. is a cranial nerve palsy
    D. is diagnostic of upper motor neuron lesion
    E. is normal

E is correct.
Avoid checking for nystagmus in the extremes of gaze, but rather where both eyes can see your finger.

1.034 Decreased deep tendon reflexes may be seen in all of the following conditions EXCEPT:
- A. neuromuscular disease
- B. lower motor neuron disease
- C. muscular disease
- D. sensory impairment
- E. upper motor neuron disease

E is correct.
Hyperreflexia is consistent with upper motor neuron disease.

1.035 A normal plantar response is:
- A. plantar flexion of toes, a negative Babinski
- B. plantar flexion of toes, a positive Babinski
- C. dorsiflexion of great toe with fanning of the others, a positive Babinski
- D. dorsiflexion of great toe with fanning of the others, a negative Babinski
- E. plantar flexion of great toe without fanning of the others, a positive Babinski

A is correct.
Better to say the plantar response is up or down.

1.036 Astereognosis is best described as:
- A. only feeling one of two simultaneous stimuli
- B. inability to recognize objects placed in hand
- C. loss of two-point discrimination
- D. loss of point localization
- E. inability to sense the position of a joint

B is correct.
Impaired with posterior column and cortical lesions.

1.037 The extraocular muscles are supplied by cranial nerves:
- A. II, III, IV
- B. III, IV, V
- C. III, IV, VI
- D. IV, V, VI
- E. IV, VI, VII

C is correct.
$LR_6(SO_4)_3$.

1.038 A patient presents with his daughter who states that her father cannot remember things. She also states she has noted a change in his personality in that he is becoming very aggressive and his speech is frequently incoherent. The MOST likely the problem with this patient is:
- A. delirium
- B. dementia
- C. TIAs
- D. alcohol withdrawal
- E. seizures

B is correct.
Memory loss and personality changes are characteristic of dementia. Medical causes should be ruled out first.

1.039 You note that your patient has an uneven smile and that the creases on the left side of the face are less prominent than on the right. However, movements of the forehead and eyebrows are symmetrical. The MOST likely diagnosis is:
- A. peripheral lesion of CN VII
- B. central lesion of CN VII
- C. peripheral lesion of CN V
- D. central lesion of CN IX

C is correct.
Presentation of lesion of the middle branch of the trigeminal nerve is described.

1.040 When examining the fundi with the hand-held ophthalmoscope, you use your:
   A. left hand with left eye to patient's right eye
   B. right hand with left eye to patient's left eye
   C. right hand with right eye to patient's left eye
   D. left hand with right eye to patient's right eye
   E. right hand with right eye to patient's right eye

E is correct.
Same hand, same eye, to same eye.

1.041 Sudden loss of resistance on muscle strength testing may indicate:
   A. pain or hysteria
   B. pain or mild weakness
   C. mild weakness or hysteria
   D. severe weakness

A is correct.
Sudden giving out is not associated with weakness.

1.042 Which location will have the best two-point discrimination?
   A. fingertip
   B. dorsum of hand
   C. dorsum of foot
   D. plantar aspect of foot
   E. anterior thigh

A is correct.
Two-point discrimination depends on the density of touch receptors.

1.043 Which statement best describes the effect of motor lesions on reflexes?
   A. upper and lower motor lesions do not affect reflexes
   B. upper and lower motor lesions decrease DTRs
   C. upper and lower motor lesions increase DTRs
   D. upper motor lesions increase DTRs and lower motor lesions decrease DTRs
   E. upper motor lesions decrease DTRs and lower motor lesions increase DTRs

D is correct.
Since upper motor neurons are inhibitory and oppose the action of lower motor neurons.

1.044 CN I assessment is indicated for the complaint of:
   A. hearing loss
   B. memory loss
   C. gait disturbance
   D. taste disturbance
   E. hemiparesis

D is correct.
Smell and taste overlap, so assessment of the olfactory nerve is indicated in patients with taste disturbances.

1.045 CN II assessment is BEST done by:
   A. gross hearing test (whisper)
   B. gross hearing test (watch tick)
   C. audiometry
   D. common odors like vanilla
   E. Snellen chart

E is correct.
Visual acuity should be assessed with a Snellen or Rosenbaum chart.

1.046 The MOST severe form of multiple sclerosis is:
   A. relapsing/remitting
   B. chronic/progressive
   C. relapsing/progressive
   D. acute/remitting

C is correct.
Designated relapsing/progressive patients have chronic progressive disease exacerbated by acute attacks and little remission.

1.047 The MOST sensitive diagnostic test for multiple sclerosis is:
- A. CSF protein
- B. MRI
- C. CT
- D. myelogram
- E. LP

B is correct.
Very sensitive, but not specific to MS, as plaques occur in Lyme disease, normal elderly patients, and uncontrolled hypertension as well.

1.048 The three cardinal motor signs of Parkinson's disease are:
- A. athetosis, bradykinesia, and chorea
- B. chorea, scissors gait, athetosis
- C. bradykinesia, chorea, and rigidity
- D. tremor (resting or postural), bradykinesia, and rigidity
- E. scissors gait, bradykinesia, and athetosis

D is correct.
Athetoid movements are associated with spasticity and cerebral palsy. Scissors gait is seen with bilateral spastic paresis and choreiform movements with (well) chorea.

1.049 Which infectious agent may be responsible for a Bell's palsy?
- A. *Escherichia coli*
- B. *Borrelia burgdorferi*
- C. *Salmonella typhi*
- D. *Chlamydia trachomatis*

B is correct.
Lyme disease, as well as agents of bacterial otitis media, may cause a facial nerve palsy.

1.050 The MOST common cause of recurrent seizures in children is:
- A. idiopathic
- B. trauma
- C. cerebrovascular
- D. drug withdrawal

A is correct.
After age 30, an underlying cause becomes more and more likely in new-onset seizures.

TEST PLAN FOR SECTION 1: NERVOUS SYSTEM

Tasks/areas assessed	Hx and PE	Dx studies	Diagnosis	Prognosis	Management Health maintenance	Clinical intervention	Clinical therapeutics	Applying scientific concepts
Total questions = 50	14	2	10	2	1	2	1	18
Diseases/disorders					*question numbers*			
Brain abscess								
Meningitis	35							
Alzheimer's disease								
Multiple sclerosis		47	38					
Parkinson's disease			48	46				
Neuralgia/neuritis	42		1					
Neuropathies	6,24,25,39		8,29					2,9,26,31,33,37,43,49
CNS trauma	32,45	19	17,18					
Transient cerebral ischemia								
Stroke					7			
Seizure			15	16		10,28		27,50
CVA	41							12,22
Neoplasms							29	
Other CNS diseases	3,14,30,34,40		4,5					11,13,20,21,36,44

SECTION 2: EYE

2.001 All of the following are risk factors for glaucoma EXCEPT:
   A. high fat diet
   B. advancing age
   C. elevated intraocular pressure
   D. family history of glaucoma
   E. African-American heritage

A is correct.
No associations with diet have been documented. All of the other factors listed increase an individual's risk of developing glaucoma.

2.002 Fine vessel injection around the border of the cornea producing a red-violet halo (ciliary flush) suggests inflammation in:
   A. lids or lacrimal apparatus
   B. palpebral conjunctiva
   C. bulbar conjunctiva or lids
   D. palpebral conjunctiva or lacrimal apparatus
   E. corneal or intraocular structures

E is correct.
Palpebral and bulbar conjunctival injection may be associated with primary conjunctivitis or inflammation of the lids or lacrimal apparatus.

2.003 Bacterial conjunctivitis:
   A. has a mucopurulent discharge
   B. exhibits seasonal recurrence
   C. has severe pain
   D. causes loss of vision
   E. is associated with URI symptoms

A is correct.
Bacterial infections result in acute local processes related to the point of entry; systemic complaints suggest viral or allergic etiologies. Severe pain is not associated with acute conjunctivitis and suggests a more serious problem. Allergic conjunctivitis frequently recurs seasonally as the precipitating allergen appears in the environment.

2.004 A 45-year-old black man presents complaining of severe pain and decreased vision in both eyes for 1 day. On exam, you note ciliary flush, essentially normal conjunctiva, and cloudiness of the cornea with fixed, mid-dilated pupils. You suspect:
   A. acute bacterial conjunctivitis
   B. allergic conjunctivitis
   C. iritis
   D. cataract
   E. acute glaucoma

E is correct.
The patient's race and age increase the risk of glaucoma. The presentation is consistent with this diagnosis. Bacterial and allergic conjunctivitis are not usually painful and do no affect the pupillary reactions. Iritis may be painful (but generally not so much as glaucoma) and may also cause ciliary flush. The pupils in iritis would be small and the cornea clear or lightly cloudy.

2.005 The person with acute glaucoma:
   A. should be referred to an ophthalmologist within a few days
   B. should be seen by an ophthalmologist within a week
   C. should be seen by an ophthalmologist now
   D. may be managed by the primary care provider
   E. may be managed by the PA with ophthalmologist telephone consultation

C is correct.
Immediate attention by an ophthalmologist is necessary for the patient with acute glaucoma. Interim therapy with acetazolamide, glycerol, and pilocarpine may be initiated in consultation with the ophthalmologist, but the patient needs to be seen.

2.006 The MOST common and usefl treatment for a subconjunctival hemorrhage without marked swelling is
    A. cycloplegic drops
    B. steroid drops
    C. antibiotic ointment
    D. reassurance
    E. steroid-antibiotic combination therapy

D is correct.
Subconjunctival hemorrhage is self-limiting in an otherwise healthy patient. None of the medications listed is indicated.

2.007 The MOST feasible method for assessing intraocular pressure in a primary care practice is:
    A. producing a crescentic shadow with a light directed across the iris
    B. applanation tonometer
    C. hand-held applanation tonometer
    D. Schiotz tonometry
    E. air-jet tonometry

D is correct.
The crescentic shadow suggests increased risk of narrow-angle glaucoma (the less common form) but does not assess intraocular pressure, which is best measured in the primary care setting with the Schiotz tonometer.

2.008 Evidence of hypertensive retinopathy on funduscopy includes all of the following EXCEPT:
    A. blurring of the optic disc
    B. A-V nicking
    C. hard exudates
    D. flame hemorrhages
    E. increased cup to greater than 1/2 disc diameter

E is correct.
Increased cupping results from increased intraocular pressure, which is characteristic of glaucoma.

2.009 A 20-year-old male who does not wear glasses or contacts presents with red eyes and blurry vision. Visual acuity done in triage is 20/40 OD, 20/40 OS, 20/40 OU. Which diagnosis is LEAST likely?
    A. conjunctivitis
    B. corneal injury/infection
    C. iritis
    D. acute narrow-angle glaucoma
    E. open-angle glaucoma

A is correct.
Conjunctivitis does not generally affect vision. The presence of documented decreased vision in this patient requires evaluation for one of these other causes of red eyes.

2.010 Painless red eye(s) suggests:
    A. conjunctivitis
    B. corneal injury/infection
    C. iritis
    D. acute glaucoma
    E. open-angle glaucoma

A is correct.
Conjunctivitis does not generally cause pain. Painful red eyes require evaluation for one of these other causes.

2.011 A 28-year-old woman with painful decreased vision and red eyes is noted to have preauricular lymphadenopathy. This suggests:
    A. herpes keratitis
    B. bacterial conjunctivitis
    C. viral conjunctivitis
    D. allergic conjunctivitis
    E. iritis

A is correct.
While the adenopathy may be associated with viral conjunctivitis, pain and decreased vision are not. Bacterial and allergic conjunctivitis is not associated with preauricular lymphadenopathy, pain, or loss of vision.

2.012 Pupils mid-dilated and fixed in a 50-year-old patient with red, painful eyes suggests:
   A. bacterial conjunctivitis
   B. viral conjunctivitis
   C. allergic conjunctivitis
   D. acute glaucoma
   E. chemical conjunctivitis

D is correct.
Conjunctivitis does not affect the pupils. Acute glaucoma characteristically presents with fixed, mid-dilated pupils.

2.013 A 40-year-old male construction worker complains of a yellow-red lesion in the nasal sclera that has begun to interfere with his vision; you diagnose:
   A. pterygium
   B. pinguecula
   C. subconjunctival hemorrhage
   D. arcus senilis
   E. episcleritis

A is correct.
A pinguecula is a nodule in the conjunctiva, usually in the nasal area, causing mild discoloration; the related lesion pterygium is vascularized and may encroach on the cornea. It is common in patients who are frequently exposed to strong sunlight. Arcus senilis is a hypopigmented ring around the iris that has no effect on vision. Episcleritis is an inflammation of the superficial vessels and does not affect vision.

2.014 The first part of the eye exam in all patients with eye complaints includes:
   A. inspection of cornea
   B. lid eversion
   C. inspection of lids
   D. visual acuity
   E. tonometry

D is correct.
Visual acuity should be assessed in all patients with eye complaints. Subtle insidious loss of vision may not be noted by patients. The exam or treatments may interfere with the assessment if done later. Documentation of intact vision is important for medical-legal reasons prior to treatment.

2.015 A pinhole test in a patient with decreased vision is to assess for:
   A. glaucoma
   B. detached retina
   C. uncorrected refractive error
   D. cataracts
   E. herpes keratitis

C is correct.
The pinhole test is useful in demonstrating uncorrected refractive error. It will not improve vision in patients with any of the other disorders listed.

2.016 Drugs useful in primary care of bacterial conjunctivitis include:
   A. erythromycin ointment, bacitracin ointment, sodium sulfacetamide
   B. neomycin ointment, bacitracin ointment, sodium sulfacetamide
   C. erythromycin ointment, bacitracin-steroid combination, sodium sulfacetamide
   D. erythromycin ointment, bacitracin ointment, Vasocon-A®
   E. neomycin ointment, bacitracin-steroid combination, Vasocon-A®

A is correct.
These drugs are generally recommended. Most authorities suggest that steroids not be used in primary care, as corneal ulcers and perforation may result. Neomycin causes allergic keratitis in 5% of patients and should be avoided. Vasocon-A® is an antihistamine-decongestant that may mask symptoms but will not treat the infection.

2.017 The Morgan Lens® is:
   A. type of soft contact lens
   B. type of hard contact lens
   C. device to assess refractive error
   D. used to irrigate eyes
   E. device used to assess color vision

D is correct.
The Morgan Lens® is a contact lens-like device with an attached irrigation line for eye irrigation.

2.018 Which of the following is NOT acceptable for removing superficial foreign bodies on the cornea?
   A. irrigation
   B. Morgan Lens®
   C. Q-tip
   D. 18-gauge needle
   E. sterile "golf-stick"

B is correct.
The Morgan Lens® should not be placed over a corneal foreign body. The other methods listed are acceptable for foreign body removal.

2.019 A 68-year-old man presents, complaining of chronic dry eyes. The MOST common cause of this condition is:
   A. foreign body
   B. infection
   C. collagen vascular disease
   D. age
   E. Sjogren's syndrome

D is correct.
While the condition may result from connective tissue disease, drug use, or neurological disease, the most common etiology is age-related physiological change.

2.020 A 20-year-old man presents with painless unilateral red eye, with mucopurulent discharge, itch, and tearing. A Gram stain of the discharge shows many "polys" with gram-negative intracellular diplococci. You would treat with:
   A. erythromycin ointment
   B. Cortisporin® (neomycin-steroid) ointment
   C. IM Rocephin®
   D. Vasocon-A®
   E. neomycin ointment without steroid

C is correct.
Polymorphonuclear leukocytes with intracellular gram-negative diplococci are presumptive of gonococcal infection, and systemic therapy with appropriate antibiotics is indicated. Traditionally, penicillin has been used, but the increased incidence of penicillinase-producing *Neisseria gonorrhoeae* (PPNG) causes many providers to prefer Rocephin® or other nonpenicillin therapy.

2.021 Emergency surgery may be necessary in which form of cataract?
   A. congenital
   B. traumatic
   C. early senile
   D. juvenile
   E. early nuclear sclerosis

B is correct.
Traumatic (and very advanced senile) cataracts may result in inflammation and glaucoma necessitating emergency surgery. Congenital and juvenile cataracts should be corrected urgently to prevent amblyopia. Early nuclear sclerosis (early senile cataract) may respond to eyeglasses alone and does not require emergency surgery.

2.022 Gram stain of a smear from a 17-year-old with conjunctivitis shows many eosinophils. This suggests:
   A. bacterial conjunctivitis
   B. viral conjunctivitis
   C. allergic conjunctivitis
   D. herpes keratoconjunctivitis
   E. chlamydial conjunctivitis

C is correct.
Polymorphonuclear leukocytes would suggest bacterial, lymphocytes would suggest viral (including herpesvirus), and scraping for inclusion bodies, if done, would indicate chlamydial disease.

2.023 A 30-year-old man presents with eye pain and decreased vision after a battery exploded in his face, while he attempted to jump-start a car. You should first:
   A. instill a cycloplegic
   B. instill an anesthetic
   C. irrigate copiously
   D. instill a steroid
   E. instill antibiotics

C is correct.
While any of the medications listed may be indicated, the FIRST thing to do would be to irrigate the eye with copious quantities of Ringer's.

2.024 A 35-year-old man presents with painful loss of vision while using a grinding wheel with no eye protection. A metallic foreign body is demonstrated in the globe by x-ray. This patient should:
- A. be protected with an eye shield and referred to ophthalmologist immediately
- B. have antibiotics instilled, patched, and followed by ophthalmologist
- C. have tetanus updated, systemic antibiotics, and followed by primary care provider
- D. have tetanus updated, topical antibiotics, and followed by ophthalmologist
- E. have antibiotics instilled, patched, and followed by primary care provider

A is correct.
Penetrating injuries to the globe should be protected with a Fox shield and seen by an ophthalmologist as an emergency. No medications should be instilled.

2.025 A well 20-year-old man presents with sudden unilateral loss of vision after a "hit" in a rugby game. This presentation is MOST likely:
- A. central retinal artery occlusion
- B. cataract
- C. glaucoma
- D. temporal arteritis
- E. detached retina

E is correct.
Central retinal artery occlusion is most commonly due to atheromatous disease, which is unlikely in this patient. Juvenile cataract would be gradual in onset and not related to trauma. Glaucoma is unlikely at this age, as is temporal arteritis.

2.026 Therapeutic intervention in acute angle-closure glaucoma may include any of the following EXCEPT:
- A. oral glycerol
- B. antibiotics for infection if glaucoma is secondary to inflammation
- C. miotic agent like pilocarpine drops
- D. acetazolamide
- E. systemic and topical steroids

E is correct.
Systemic and topical steroids increase intraocular pressure and could exacerbate acute angle-closure glaucoma. All of the other medications listed may be used.

2.027 Agents used in the management of chronic open-angle glaucoma include:
- A. cholinergics, anticholinesterases, sympathomimetics, and β-blockers
- B. anticholinergics, cholinesterases, sympathomimetics, and β-blockers
- C. cholinergics, cholinesterases, α-blockers, and beta-agonists
- D. anticholinergics, anticholinesterases, α-blockers, and beta-agonists
- E. anticholinergics, anticholinesterases, sympathomimetics, and β-blockers

A is correct.
Cholinergics like pilocarpine facilitate outflow of aqueous by contraction of the ciliary body. Anticholinesterases like echothiophate iodide (Phospholine Iodide®) increase endogenous cholinergic effects. Sympathomimetics like epinephrine decrease aqueous production and possibly outflow. β-Blockers such as timolol decrease aqueous production.

2.028 When conducting a cover-uncover test on a 5-year-old, you note no movement when the right eye is covered/uncovered but lateral movement of the right eye when the left is covered and medial movement when the cover is removed. This represents:
- A. monocular left esotropia
- B. monocular right esotropia
- C. binocular exotropia
- D. monocular left exotropia
- E. monocular right exotropia

B is correct.
In the test described, the medially deviated suppressed eye moves to focus when the view of the dominant eye is covered and moves back to its abnormal position when the dominant eye is uncovered.

2.029 A neurological lesion resulting in a blind right eye with normal left vision would occur at the level of the:
  A. right optic nerve
  B. optic chiasm
  C. right optic tract
  D. right optic radiation
  E. left optic radiation

A is correct.
Lesions above the level of the optic nerve affect vision in both eyes to some degree.

2.030 Which of the following have all been shown to be helpful in preventing the progression of diabetic retinopathy?
  A. tight glycemic control, control of hypertension, cessation of smoking
  B. tight glycemic control, control of hypertension,
  C. control of hypertension, cessation of smoking
  D. tight glycemic control, cessation of smoking
  E. aspirin, control of hypertension, cessation of smoking

A is correct.
All of these help to prevent the progression of diabetic retinopathy. Aspirin has not been shown to be effective for this use.

TEST PLAN FOR SECTION 2: EYE

Tasks/areas assessed	Hx and PE	Dx studies	Diagnosis	Prognosis	Management			Applying scientific concepts
					Health maintenance	Clinical intervention	Clinical therapeutics	
Total questions = 30	1	5	5	0	0	3	6	10
					question numbers			
Diseases/disorders								
Blurred vision/decreased acuity		14,15	13					25
Cataract							21	
Diabetic retinopathy								30
Diseases of globe, retinal detachment/puncture								
Glaucoma	1	7	4,12				26,27	5
Hypersensitivity retinopathy			8					
Blunt and penetrating trauma						6,24	17,19	
Conjunctivitis		9,22	11			23	16	2, 3,10,20
Disorders of optic nerve/visual path								29
Strabismus								28
Other diseases of lids and lacrimal system								18

SECTION 3: EAR, NOSE, MOUTH, AND THROAT

3.001 In oral cancer screening, which lesions are MOST likely premalignant?
    A. red hyperplastic (erythroplasia)
    B. white patches (leukoplakia)
    C. petechial lesions of the palate
    D. those adjacent to jagged teeth
    E. swelling beneath normal-appearing mucosa

A is correct.
The predominant color in premalignant or early malignant lesions is red. White lesions are suspicious and require evaluation, but fewer of them are determined to be malignant. Petechial lesions of the palate have numerous non-neoplastic causes, including mononucleosis and vomiting. Lesions adjacent to jagged teeth or associated with loose or poorly fitted dentures are likely to be traumatic. Swellings beneath normal mucosa require evaluation but have numerous benign causes.

3.002 Which of the following all represent causes of conductive hearing loss?
    A. noise, exostoses, glomus tumors
    B. otosclerosis, drugs, acoustic neuroma
    C. otosclerosis, Meniere's disease, glomus tumors
    D. presbycusis, exostoses, noise
    E. otosclerosis, exostoses, glomus tumors

E is correct.
Otosclerosis, exostoses, and glomus tumors result in conductive hearing loss. Noise- or drug-induced loss, acoustic neuromas, Meniere's disease, and presbycusis result in sensorineural hearing loss.

3.003 A patient presents with decreased hearing acuity on the left. The Weber test refers to the left, and the Rinne demonstrates AC > BC in both ears. What is the patient's type of loss?
    A. sensorineural on the right
    B. conductive on the right
    C. sensorineural on the left
    D. conductive on the left

C is correct
In unilateral sensorineural hearing loss, air conduction remains greater than bone conduction, and the Weber test will refer to the affected ear.

3.004 An air-bone gap on audiogram is consistent with:
    A. normal hearing
    B. loss of speech discrimination
    C. conductive hearing loss
    D. sensorineural hearing loss
    E. diminished speech reception threshold

C is correct.
The air-bone gap demonstrates that sound is conducted better through the bone of the mastoid process than the auditory conduction system, thereby demonstrating pathology in the conduction system. Patients with normal hearing or sensorineural loss will not exhibit an air-bone gap on audiogram. Speech discrimination and speech reception threshold are assessed separately from the audiogram by presenting spoken words for the patient to identify.

3.005 Patients with epistaxis who require immediate
ENT referral include those requiring:
    A. any nasal packing
    B. silver nitrate cautery
    C. phenylephrine or oxymetazoline
    D. posterior nasal packing
    E. oxidized surgical cellulose

D is correct.
Patients with bleeds requiring posterior
packing have a high rate of complications and
require ENT referral. The other modalities are
commonly used by primary providers for
outpatients.

3.006 A patient with facial pain aggravated by ingestion
of hot, cold, or sweet foods who has no fever or facial
swelling suggests:
    A. temporomandibular joint dysfunction
    B. trigeminal neuralgia
    C. acute sinusitis
    D. periapical abscess
    E. caries

E is correct.
Patients with TMJ dysfunction or trigeminal
neuralgia will not have symptoms related to
the temperature of contacting substances.
Periapical abscess is aggravated by heat but
relieved by cold. Sinusitis is not aggravated by
specific foods and may have swelling and
fever.

3.007 Patients with acute laryngitis:
    A. require voice rest
    B. require empirical antibiotic therapy
    C. may benefit from topical steroids if infectious
       etiology
    D. should avoid sialogogues
    E. should reduce environmental humidity

A is correct.
Antibiotics are not indicated unless a
documented bacterial infection exists and
topical steroids are of benefit for allergic
etiologies. Sialogogues and increased
environmental humidity may be helpful.

3.008 Which of the following is true regarding tinnitus?
    A. most cases have an identifiable etiology
    B. most cases result from the same etiologies as
       hearing loss
    C. most cases do not require careful evaluation, as
       causes are benign but not treatable
    D. all patients with tinnitus should be screened for
       liver disease
    E. tinnitus often accompanies conductive but not
       sensorineural hearing loss

B is correct.
Most cases of tinnitus result from conditions
leading to some form of hearing loss. It is not
specific to conductive versus sensorineural,
and, despite this, as many as 50% of cases in
otological practice are of unknown etiology.
All cases require careful evaluation, especially
when associated with conductive hearing loss,
as serious, treatable causes are found. Liver
disease is not associated with tinnitus.

3.009 The MOST common organisms in acute otitis
media (OM) are:
    A. *Pseudomonas aeruginosa, Haemophilus
       influenzae, Moraxella catarrhalis, Staphylococcus
       epidermidis*
    B. *Streptococcus pneumoniae, H. influenzae, M.
       catarrhalis, P. aeruginosa*
    C. *S. pneumoniae, H. influenzae, M. catarrhalis,*
       enteric gram-negatives
    D. *S. pneumoniae, H. influenzae, M. catarrhalis, S.
       epidermidis*
    E. *S. pneumoniae, H. influenzae,* fungi, enteric gram-
       negatives

D is correct.
Pseudomonas and enteric gram-negatives
become important in chronic OM, and fungi
are important causative agents in otitis externa.

3.010 Treatment for acute OM may include any of the following EXCEPT:
   A. antibiotics
   B. analgesics
   C. antihistamines
   D. decongestants
   E. myringotomy

C is correct.
Antihistamines should not be used in these patients, as they may thicken secretions in the ear and interfere with drainage. Antibiotics for infection, analgesics for pain, and decongestants to promote drainage are routine therapy. Referral for myringotomy may be indicated if pain is intractable or progressive hearing loss or early mastoiditis develops, or if response to routine therapy is poor.

3.011 A good first-choice antibiotic for OM in children is:
   A. penicillin
   B. erythromycin
   C. amoxcillin/clavulanate (Augmentin®)
   D. amoxicillin
   E. cefaclor (Ceclor®)

D is correct.
Penicillin may suffice in adults but lacks coverage for *H. influenzae* (common in pediatric OM). Erythromycin alone lacks adequate coverage, so in children allergic to penicillin it is used in conjunction with sulfa (Pediazole®). Augmentin® and Ceclor® are usually reserved as second-line drugs due to their broad spectrum of activity and higher cost.

3.012 A 50-year-old, diabetic man presents with painful swollen-shut ear canal and exquisitely tender pinna and tragus. He has swollen preauricular nodes and a temperature of 101°F. There is a greenish, sweet-smelling discharge from the ear. You would:
   A. treat with analgesics and topical neomycin-polymyxin
   B. treat with analgesics, topical neomycin-polymyxin, and oral systemic antibiotic
   C. treat with analgesics and oral systemic antibiotic
   D. treat with analgesics, oral systemic antibiotic, and decongestants
   E. refer the patient to a otorhinolaryngologist

E is correct.
The scenario suggests malignant otitis externa—a rare but life-threatening infection in diabetics caused by *P. aeruginosa* that requires hospitalization and parenteral antibiotics.

3.013 Which is FALSE regarding sinusitis:
   A. viral sinusitis is a common, self-limited component of the common cold
   B. rhinorrhea and nasal stuffiness are nonspecific symptoms of sinusitis
   C. acute purulent bacterial sinusitis is a common sequela of the common cold
   D. allergic or vasomotor rhinitis may be an antecedent to acute bacterial sinusitis
   E. systemic diseases like cystic fibrosis may contribute to acute sinusitis

C is correct.
Only 0.5–5% of patients will develop acute bacterial sinusitis, while viral sinusitis is commonly associated with the common cold. Predisposing factors for acute bacterial sinusitis may include allergy, vasomotor rhinitis, or occasionally systemic diseases like cystic fibrosis or Kartagener's syndrome.

3.014 Common bacterial causes of acute sinusitis include:
   A. *P. aeruginosa, H. influenzae, S. epidermidis*
   B. *S. pneumoniae, H. influenzae, P. aeruginosa*
   C. *H. influenzae, M. catarrhalis*, enteric gram-negatives
   D. streptococci, *H. influenzae, M. catarrhalis*
   E. pneumococci, *H. influenzae*, enteric gram-negatives

D is correct.
Common causative organisms are similar to those for acute OM.

3.015 The MOST important therapy in all patients with acute purulent sinusitis is:
  A. decongestants
  B. antihistamines
  C. antibiotics
  D. analgesics
  E. steroids

A is correct.
Although most providers will also use antibiotics in mild disease, close to 50% of patients may be cured with decongestants alone; more severe disease (toxic, febrile, failing decongestants, or with complications) will require antibiotics. Analgesics may be required for some patients. Antihistamines may be useful if an underlying allergic component exists. Steroids are of little benefit and may impair the patient's response to infection.

3.016 Which is FALSE regarding antibiotic therapy of streptococcal pharyngitis?
  A. reduces severity of symptoms
  B. reduces duration of symptoms
  C. prevents acute rheumatic fever
  D. prevents acute glomerulonephritis
  E. reduces the contagious period

D is correct.
While treatment of strep (usually pen VK) is effective for each of the other choices, it does not prevent poststreptococcal AGN.

3.017 Splenomegaly in a patient with pharyngitis suggests:
  A. gonococcal infection
  B. diphtheria
  C. Epstein-Barr virus
  D. Coxsackie A virus
  E. group A beta-hemolytic strep (*S. pyogenes*)

C is correct.
All of these are causative agents in acute pharyngitis, but only EBV (the causative agent of infectious mononucleosis) is associated with splenomegaly (about 50% of patients).

3.018 A 21-year-old woman presents to your clinic with pharyngitis, fever, tonsillar exudates, and anterior cervical adenopathy for 2 days. She denies any exposure to strep, a history of rheumatic fever or mononucleosis, and any ongoing medical problems. She is taking oral contraceptives (OCs) and denies any allergies to medications. She is sexually active with several partners but denies missed pills and has successfully used OCs for 1 year. She admits to orogenital contact and denies any vaginal discharge, dyspareunia, abdominal complaints, or known contacts with sexually transmitted diseases. Laboratory diagnosis for this patient should include all of the following EXCEPT:
  A. rapid strep-antigen test
  B. throat culture if negative rapid strep
  C. wet prep if cheesy-appearing pharyngeal exudates
  D. throat culture on Thayer-Martin medium
  E. monospot or heterophile antibody titer

E is correct.
Testing for mononucleosis is not indicated due to the short duration of symptoms. Neither the monospot nor the heterophile would be reactive at this time. Rapid strep followed by throat culture if negative is indicated to rule out *S. pyogenes* infection. If the pharyngeal exudate is cheesy in appearance, a wet prep will identify *Candida*. The history of orogenital contact requires that *N. gonorrhoeae* be considered as a possible cause, necessitating the Thayer-Martin culture medium.

3.019 Rare but potentially lethal cardiac rhythm disturbances have been observed in patients taking the second-generation antihistamines terfenadine (Seldane®; withdrawn from market) or astemizole (Hismanal®) concurrently with:
  A. penicillin
  B. erythromycin
  C. tetracycline
  D. amoxicillin
  E. ampicillin

B is correct.
This has also been seen with concomitant ketoconazole, an oral antifungal.

3.020 A Gram stain of nasal secretions in allergic rhinitis would likely show many:
  A. polymorphonuclear leukocytes with intracellular gram-negative diplococci
  B. lymphocytes
  C. eosinophils
  D. polymorphonuclear leukocytes
  E. large gram-positive football-shaped organisms

C is correct.
"Polys" are associated with bacterial infection in general, and if found with gram-negative intracellular diplococci, they might suggest *M. catarrhalis* or *Neisseria* infection. Lymphocytes suggest viral etiologies, and gram-positive "footballs" are likely to be *Candida*.

3.021 Epiglottitis in an unimmunized child is MOST likely caused by:
  A. respiratory syncytial virus (RSV)
  B. *H. influenzae* type b (HIB)
  C. rotavirus
  D. influenza virus A
  E. influenza virus B

B is correct.
Epiglottitis is an acute bacterial infection of the epiglottis, with HIB the predominant organism in unimmunized children. (The other organisms are all viral.)

3.022 A 46-year-old woman comes to the ER because she has a grasshopper in her left ear. Appropriate interventions include all of the following EXCEPT:
  A. drown the insect in water or oil
  B. irrigate canal with water to flush insect out
  C. remove with wax curette
  D. use wall suction to remove insect
  E. inquire as to how it got there

D is correct.
All of the other interventions listed are appropriate. However, wall suction should not be used in the ear.

3.023 The MOST common presenting symptom of laryngeal carcinoma is:
  A. dysphagia
  B. lymphadenopathy
  C. airway obstruction
  D. hoarseness
  E. sore throat

D is correct.
Laryngeal carcinoma most commonly presents with painless hoarse voice in a smoker. Airway obstruction, dysphagia, and lymphadenopathy are possible, but later in the disease process.

3.024 Findings of otitis externa (OE) may include any of the following EXCEPT:
  A. ear pain and itching
  B. edema of the canal
  C. diminished hearing
  D. serous fluid behind tympanic membrane
  E. foul-smelling discharge

D is correct.
Serous fluid behind the TM is found with serous otitis media; the other findings are consistent with OE.

3.025 Treatment of viral pharyngitis may include any of the following EXCEPT:
A. acetaminophen
B. saline gargles
C. erythromycin 250 mg PO QID × 10d
D. increased fluid intake and rest
E. ibuprofen

C is correct.
Antibiotics are not indicated in viral pharyngitis. It is a self-limited disease, and only comfort measures are needed.

3.026 The MOST frequent cause of nosebleeds is:
A. granulomatous disease
B. neoplasm
C. hypertension
D. local trauma
E. coagulopathy

D is correct.
Local trauma to Kisselbach's area of the nasal septum, especially when associated with dry environments, is the etiology of most epistaxis. Hypertension per se is not a cause of epistaxis. The other choices may cause epistaxis, but much less often.

3.027 The MOST common class of etiologic agents for upper respiratory tract infections in children is:
A. mycoplasmal
B. viral
C. bacterial
D. fungal
E. parasitic

B is correct.
The vast majority of all URIs are viral.

3.028 Which of the following statements is true about acute OM?
A. patients will complain of ear pain with associated fever, and decreased hearing
B. OM may cause acute sensorineural hearing loss
C. in adults the length of the eustachian tube increases the incidence of the disease
D. the infection cannot spread to the subdural space
E. the infection cannot spread to the mastoid

A is correct.
This describes the typical presentation. Hearing impairment in acute OM is usually conductive due to fluid accumulation. Shorter, straighter eustachian tubes in children make them more prone to the disease, and infection may spread to the mastoid or even the subdural space.

3.029 Clear, watery nasal discharge, sneezing, and itchy, watery eyes suggest:
A. sinusitis
B. allergic rhinitis
C. viral URI
D. vasomotor rhinitis
E. cocaine abuse

B is correct.
Sinusitis more commonly produces a mucoid or mucopurulent discharge with nasal congestion, facial pressure, or pain the predominant complaints. Viral URI complaints are similar to sinusitis, but without the facial pain. Fever may be a component of both of these. Vasomotor rhinitis generally relates to some specific recurring exposure, such as to cold air or exercise, and, like cocaine abuse, lacks the eye components of the given history.

3.030 Which of the following is MORE suggestive of allergic rhinitis than the common cold:
A. itching
B. fever
C. postnasal drip
D. seasonal history
E. sneezing

D is correct.
A clear history of seasonal recurrence is the most specific distinction between these two.

3.031 Which of the following are useful in the prophylactic treatment of allergic rhinitis?
    A. oral decongestants, intranasal steroids, cromolyn sodium, and immunotherapy
    B. avoidance, oral steroids, cromolyn sodium, and immunotherapy
    C. decongestant sprays, intranasal steroids, cromolyn sodium, and immunotherapy
    D. avoidance, intranasal steroids, cromolyn sodium, and immunotherapy
    E. avoidance, intranasal steroids, antihistamines, and decongestant sprays

D is correct.
Antihistamines and decongestants are best used symptomatically. Steroids may prevent and limit the allergic response. The other modalities are only helpful in preventing the allergic response.

3.032 Cocaine's effects on the nasal septum may include:
    A. vasoconstriction, anesthesia, necrosis, perforation
    B. vasoconstriction, hyperesthesia, necrosis, perforation
    C. vasoconstriction, anesthesia, hyperplasia
    D. vasodilatation, anesthesia, perforation
    E. vasodilatation, anesthesia, necrosis

A is correct.
Cocaine is used therapeutically for its vasoconstrictor and anesthetic effects on nasal mucosa. However, abuse of the drug leads to necrosis and perforation of the nasal septum.

3.033 A 28-year-old man presents, complaining of pain in left maxillary area for 3 days, which he believes is his sinuses. This pain is aggravated by heat and relieved with ice packs. You suspect an abscessed tooth. Which technique is MOST diagnostic?
    A. palpation for mobility of the tooth
    B. soft tissue palpation of the gums for fluctuance
    C. tooth percussion for tenderness
    D. inspection for decay
    E. lymph node palpation

C is correct.
Tapping the suspected tooth with a tongue blade or butt end of a dental mirror will produce pain in an abscessed tooth, but not in maxillary sinusitis. The gums and teeth may appear normal.

3.034 A 50-year-old man presents, complaining of stabbing pain in the left maxillary area for 3 days, which he believes is his sinuses. This pain is unrelated to temperature or type of food, and he denies fever, nasal congestion, discharge, or swelling. You suspect:
    A. trigeminal neuralgia
    B. caries
    C. abscess
    D. sialadenitis
    E. parotitis

A is correct.
The character and location of the pain and age of the patient are consistent with trigeminal neuralgia. The absence of fever, nasal congestion, discharge, and swelling argue against sinusitis The lack of reaction to temperature argues against caries, abscesses, and sialadenitis. Parotitis is unlikely at this age and would result in facial swelling.

3.035 Comfort measures for patients with sinusitis may include:
    A. elevate foot of bed, dehumidifiers, inhaled steam, fluid restriction
    B. elevate head of bed, dehumidifiers, inhaled steam, fluid restriction
    C. elevate head of bed, humidifiers, inhaled steam, encourage fluid
    D. elevate foot of bed, dehumidifiers, fluid restriction
    E. elevate foot of bed, dehumidifiers, inhaled steam

C is correct.
These measures all thin secretions and promote drainage.

3.036 Warning signs of complications of acute sinusitis may include:
  A. purulent nasal discharge, pain increased leaning forward
  B. high fever, lid edema, proptosis
  C. toothache, opacity on transillumination
  D. thickened mucosa on x-ray, positive nasal culture
  E. air-fluid levels on x-ray, tenderness to percussion

B is correct.
These findings, particularly in a "toxic" appearing patient, suggest retrograde extension of the infection along venous channels.

3.037 An 18-month-old presents with inspiratory stridor, barking cough, and low-grade fever. You suspect:
  A. epiglottitis
  B. supraglottitis
  C. viral laryngotracheobronchitis
  D. bacterial bronchitis
  E. pneumonia

C is correct.
Supraglottitis and epiglottitis are usually bacterial and acute in onset with severe sore throat and high fever. Cough (vs. stridor, which suggests upper airway obstruction) is predominant in bronchitis and pneumonia.

3.038 Which of the following is FALSE regarding epiglottitis?
  A. patients appear acutely ill
  B. sudden onset of severe sore throat is common
  C. high fever is common
  D. pooling, drooling, and tripod posturing is exhibited
  E. indirect laryngoscopy should be used to confirm diagnosis

E is correct.
Indirect laryngoscopy in the patient with epiglottitis is likely to precipitate laryngospasm and total airway obstruction. Lateral soft tissue x-ray may confirm the diagnosis.

3.039 X-ray findings in croup and epiglottitis include:
  A. thumb sign in both
  B. thumb sign in croup, steeple sign in epiglottitis
  C. thumb sign in epiglottitis, steeple sign in croup
  D. steeple sign in both
  E. thumb sign in croup only, steeple sign in epiglottitis or croup

C is correct.
The thumb sign in epiglottitis represents the swollen enlarged epiglottis seen in the lateral view; it is not seen in croup. The steeple sign in croup is the church-steeple appearance of the air column in the trachea due to subglottic narrowing. In epiglottitis, obstruction results in widening of the subglottic air column.

3.040 In evaluation of a patient after an episode of spontaneous, self-limited, posterior epistaxis, you find a history of chronic sinus infection and opacified sinuses on x-ray. You should:
  A. aggressively treat the sinuses with antibiotics and decongestants; follow in 2 weeks, sooner PRN
  B. treat the sinuses symptomatically only; follow in 2–4 weeks, sooner PRN
  C. not treat the sinuses and educate the patient regarding home care of epistaxis; follow PRN
  D. treat the sinuses with 2 weeks of antibiotics and decongestants; educate regarding epistaxis; follow PRN
  E. refer for ENT evaluation

E is correct.
Malignancy must be ruled out in this patient.

3.041 Laboratory evaluation in a patient with severe acute epistaxis may include:
- A. CBC, PT, PTT, bleeding time, type and screen/crossmatch
- B. CBC, electrolytes, BUN, creatinine
- C. PT, PTT, BUN, creatinine
- D. H/H, platelets, bleeding time, type and screen/crossmatch
- E. electrolytes, BUN, glucose, UA

A is correct.
Electrolytes, BUN, glucose, creatinine, and urinalysis are unnecessary and do not add to the data base. Patients with epistaxis need to be assessed for blood loss (H/H), clotting abilities (platelets, PT/PTT, bleeding time) and blood transfusion (type and screen/crossmatch).

3.042 A side effect of meperidine (Demerol®) of particular concern in the patient with significant epistaxis is:
- A. sedation
- B. analgesia
- C. hypertension
- D. hypotension
- E. respiratory depression

D is correct.
In a patient who may already be volume-depleted, the side effect of hypotension is particularly worrisome.

3.043 A toddler presents with audible high-pitched inspiratory and expiratory sounds, diminished breath sounds on the left side, rhinorrhea, and a temperature of 99°F (tympanic). The mother states he has been well until today. You suspect:
- A. croup
- B. epiglottitis
- C. bronchitis
- D. foreign body
- E. pneumonia

D is correct.
Stridorous respirations in a well toddler should suggest trauma rather than illness, especially aspirated foreign body. If the object is small enough to pass the glottic opening, it is more likely to enter the right mainstem bronchus and obstruct the right side, hence the diminished sounds on the right only.

3.044 An 18-year-old otherwise healthy patient presents with acute pharyngitis. You should:
- A. treat symptomatically pending throat culture results
- B. treat symptomatically, give 2 days of antibiotics pending TC result
- C. treat symptomatically only, follow PRN
- D. treat symptomatically, give 7 days of antibiotics
- E. give 10 days of antibiotics, advise OTC medications PRN

A is correct.
The vast majority of these cases will be viral; therefore, unless extenuating circumstances exist, antibiotics are not indicated. In many settings, you will be able to do a rapid strep test, with treating or not treating based on the results.

3.045 An 18-year-old otherwise healthy woman presents with acute pharyngitis. She states her roommate was diagnosed with "strep." You should:
- A. treat symptomatically pending throat culture results
- B. treat symptomatically, give 2 days of antibiotics pending TC results
- C. treat symptomatically only, follow PRN
- D. treat symptomatically, give 7 days of antibiotics
- E. give 10 days of antibiotics, advise OTC medications PRN

E is correct.
The history of close contact with a documented case of strep justifies treatment with antibiotics. Since strep tests and throat cultures lack 100% sensitivity and treatment is inexpensive and benign, it makes sense to complete the full 10 days for rheumatic fever (RF) prophylaxis.

3.046 An 18-year-old patient with a history of rheumatic fever presents with acute pharyngitis. You should:
  A. treat symptomatically pending throat culture results
  B. treat symptomatically, give 2 days of antibiotics pending TC results
  C. treat symptomatically only, follow PRN
  D. treat symptomatically, give 7 days of antibiotics
  E. give 10 days of antibiotics, advise OTC medications PRN

E is correct.
This patient's history of prior RF mandates a more aggressive approach to pharyngitis.

3.047 Foreign-body maneuvers used in infants include:
  A. back-blows, Heimlich maneuvers, direct laryngoscopy
  B. back-blows, chest thrusts, blind finger probes
  C. blind finger probes, chest thrusts, direct laryngoscopy
  D. back-blows, chest thrusts, Heimlich maneuvers
  E. back-blows, chest thrusts, direct laryngoscopy

E is correct.
According to the American Heart Association criteria, blind finger probes and Heimlich maneuvers are not used in infants with foreign-body airway obstruction.

3.048 Cancers of the oral cavity:
  A. cause extreme pain in their early stages
  B. seldom metastasize before being diagnosed
  C. are highly correlated with tobacco use
  D. are not associated with alcohol use
  E. have peak incidence in males in 20s, females in 30s

C is correct.
Cancers of the oral cavity are associated with tobacco and alcohol use. They present as painless lesions, and half have metastasized prior to diagnosis. The peak incidence for women is in the sixth decade, and in men it reaches and sustains a maximum at age 50.

3.049 Sensorineural hearing loss may result from pathology in the:
  A. tympanic membrane
  B. ossicle chain
  C. auditory canal
  D. cochlea
  E. malleus

D is correct.
Pathology of the auditory canal, TM, malleus, and ossicle chain interferes with the conduction of sound vibrations, i.e., a conductive hearing loss.

3.050 Most cases of strep pharyngitis can be distinguished from viral causes:
  A. by presence of petechiae
  B. by presence of exudates
  C. by presence of palatal edema
  D. by tender enlarged lymph nodes
  E. only by culture

E is correct.
There is no clinical manifestation or combination of findings that reliably distinguishes strep pharyngitis. Culture is still the "gold standard."

3.051 Proven strep pharyngitis in a patient with no drug allergies is treated with:
  A. pen VK 250 mg PO QID × 10 days   = 1000mg QD   ×10.d
  B. erythromycin 250 mg PO QID × 10 days
  C. pen VK 500 mg PO QID × 10 days
  D. pen VK 250 mg PO TID × 10 days
  E. pen VK 250 mg PO QID × 14 days

A is correct.
American Heart Association recommends this regimen in the nonpenicillin-allergic patient.

3.052 You treat a 24-year-old man for acute strep pharyngitis with 10 days of erythromycin 250 mg QID. On day 9 of treatment, he calls, stating in a muffled voice, "I am running a fever of 101 today. What should I do?" You advise:

    A. apropriate measures for fever and pain control, follow-up in office tomorrow if still febrile

    B. appropriate measures for fever and pain control, follow-up in office tomorrow regardless

    C. appropriate measures for fever and pain control, phone in 7 more days of erythromycin

    D. coming in to office for evaluation immediately if fever exceeds 103°F

    E. coming in to office for evaluation immediately

E is correct.
Fever in a compliant patient on antibiotics for 9 days mandates immediate evaluation.

3.053 When you next see the patient, he has bilateral cervical and axially lymphadenopathy, as well as a maculopapular rash. His pharynx exhibits 3+ tonsils with foul-smelling exudates. You suspect:

    A. resistant strep pharyngitis with drug rash

    B. peritonsillar abscess and septicemia

    C. mononucleosis

    D. scarlet fever

    E. varicella

C is correct.
Resistant strep is rare and would not account for the lymphadenopathy, as well as requiring a second diagnosis to account for the rash. Peritonsillar abscess and septicemia, while possible, would not account for the pattern of lymphadenopathy and has a characteristic unilateral swelling involving the soft palate on the affected side. Scarlet fever is unlikely with the antibiotics and does not explain the pharyngeal findings. The rash of chicken pox is characteristically vesicular on an erythematous base and is not associated with the lymphadenopathy or pharyngitis, as is mono.

3.054 In evaluation of a patient with hoarseness, indirect laryngoscopy:

    A. is mandatory in all patients

    B. is mandatory in all pediatric patients

    C. is mandatory in all adult smokers

    D. is mandatory in all adults

    E. is mandatory after 2–3 weeks of symptoms

E is correct.
Persistent hoarseness suggests laryngeal pathology, which can frequently be diagnosed by indirect laryngoscopy. Since hoarseness is a nonspecific symptom of the ubiquitous URI and allergy, it is reasonable not to perform immediate laryngoscopy in every patient with the complaint.

3.055 Patients with recurring cerumen impaction may be advised to:

    A. use wax remover drops (e.g., Debrox®) monthly

    B. use Q-tip to clean ear canal

    C. use ear curette to clean canal

    D. instill antifungal drops prophylactically

    E. irrigate ear canal daily with water

A is correct.
Patients should not attempt to curette the ear canal or insert Q-tips due to the risk of injury. Fungal prophylaxis is not indicated. Daily irrigation would likely result in otitis externa. Cerumen-softening drops used monthly should facilitate the natural flow of cerumen without causing significant irritation.

3.056 A well-appearing 16-year-old male with ear pain for 1 day, no fever, and no URI complaints has significant increase in pain with traction on the pinna. This suggests:
   A. otitis media
   B. serous otitis media
   C. chronic otitis media
   D. otitis externa
   E. mastoiditis

D is correct.
OM is likely to be associated with some other URI complaints. Patients with mastoiditis are ill, usually febrile, and have had OM complaints prior to developing the mastoiditis.

3.057 The MOST common cause of vertigo is:
   A. cardiac dysrhythmia
   B. labyrinthitis
   C. tumor
   D. transient ischemic attack
   E. hypotension

B is correct.
True vertigo, as opposed to dizziness or lightheadedness, is most often related to disorders of the middle ear, rather than being cardiac or neurological in origin.

3.058 A 24-year-old female presents complains of recurrent vesicular lesions on an erythematous base at the right side of her mouth, which she describes as "cold sores." The lesions present with a prodromal irritation at the site, have appeared "every time she gets a cold," and last 12–15 days regardless of anything she has tried, including antibiotic ointments, antifungal creams, steroids, moisturizers, and drying agents. She is otherwise well, takes no medications except oral contraceptives, and has no known allergies. Your diagnosis is:
   A. tinea corporis
   B. Coxsackie virus
   C. eczema
   D. herpes simplex
   E. zoster

D is correct.
The appearance of the lesions is inconsistent with tinea, as is the lack of response to antifungals. Coxsackie virus causes lesions in the mouth and on the hands and feet; it also should not be recurrent. Eczema, while recurrent, does not usually occur in this location and should be steroid responsive. Zoster (shingles) tends to be painful, follow a dermatomal distribution, and is not common in young patients.

3.059 Which of the following is NOT a possible cause of chronic or recurrent nasal congestion?
   A. allergies
   B. abuse of nose drops
   C. hyperthyroidism
   D. sarcoidosis
   E. pregnancy

C is correct.
Hypothyroidism is a possible cause, as are all of the other choices.

3.060 Chronic sinusitis is present when symptoms persist:
   A. after a single course of antibiotics
   B. annually for 1 week every 3 years
   C. more than 6 months
   D. for 1 week during two different seasons
   E. for more than 3 months

E is correct.
Chronic versus recurrent sinusitis is said to exist when symptoms persist for more than 3 months. The bacteriology of chronic sinusitis differs from acute sinusitis and necessitates different antibiotics and longer courses of treatment.

TEST PLAN FOR SECTION 3: EAR, NOSE, MOUTH, AND THROAT

Tasks/areas assessed	Hx and PE	Dx studies	Diagnosis	Prognosis	Management			Applying scientific concepts
					Health maintenance	Clinical intervention	Clinical therapeutics	
Total questions = 60	2	7	16	1	2	4	11	17
					question numbers			
Diseases/disorders								
Hearing impairment	3							2,4,8,49
Impacted cerumen					55	22		
Otitis externa			24,46			12		
Otitis media							10,11	9,28
Vertigo			57					
Other diseases of ear/mastoid								32
Acute sinusitis			6,33,34				15	13,14
Allergic rhinitis		20	29				19,31	
Bacterial/viral pharyngitis	17	18,50	53	16	51		25,44,56	45,52
Chronic rhinitis			59					
Chronic sinusitis			60				35	
Epiglottitis		36,39	37,38,43			47		21
Epistaxis		41				5	42	26
Upper respiratory infection		54	30				7	27
Herpes simplex			58					
Neoplasms			23					1,40,48

SECTION 4: RESPIRATORY SYSTEM

4.001 A patient reports that he has smoked 1½ packs of cigarettes per day for the last 20 years. How many pack-years is this?

A. 20 pack-years
B. 21.5 pack-years
C. 25 pack-years
D. 30 pack-years
E. 40 pack-years

D is correct.

PPD × years = pack-years (the best way to quantify past smoking history). You should also state current consumption and time since quitting (if applicable) to be complete.

4.002 Your patient describes episodes of sudden shortness of breath that awaken him from sleep, causing him to go to the window in order to catch his breath. This is called:

A. orthopnea
B. paroxysmal nocturnal dyspnea
C. emphysema
D. dyspnea
E. claudication

B is correct.
Associated with congestive heart failure, this represents early pulmonary edema.

4.003 Your patient describes shortness of breath when lying down and the necessity to sleep with a number of pillows or in a semisitting state. This symptom is referred to as:

A. orthopnea
B. paroxysmal nocturnal dyspnea
C. congestive heart failure
D. chronic obstructive pulmonary disease
E. reflux

A is correct.
Peripheral edema fluid returning to the central circulation causes pulmonary edema and dyspnea.

4.004 The etiology may be hemothorax if percussion of the chest wall on the side with diminished breath sounds is:

A. dull
B. resonant
C. hyperresonant
D. tympanic

A is correct.
Percussion over fluid-filled areas should be dull.

4.005 The etiology may be tension pneumothorax if percussion of the chest wall on the side with diminished breath sounds is:

A. dull
B. resonant
C. hyperresonant
D. equal to the unaffected side

C is correct.
As air accumulates under pressure, the normally resonant lung fields become hyperresonant.

4.006 This type of breath sound will MOST frequently be heard over the 1st and 2nd intercostal spaces along the sternal border:
 A. vesicular
 B. bronchovesicular
 C. bronchial
 D. tracheal

C is correct.
Higher-pitched and louder than vesicular sounds, these are normal in this area but should not be heard over the distal lung fields.

4.007 This type of breath sound has an expiratory phase that is shorter than its inspiratory phase:
 A. vesicular
 B. bronchovesicular
 C. bronchial
 D. tracheal

A is correct.
If the expiratory phase of vesicular breath sounds exceeds the inspiratory phase, then obstructive disease, such as asthma, should be suspected.

4.008 In a patient with lobar pneumonia, which of the following signs would you NOT expect to find?
 A. crackles over involved area
 B. on egophony, the "ee" sound changes to "ay"
 C. percussion will be hyperresonant over involved area
 D. vocal fremitus will be increased and clearer over involved area

C is correct.
The area of consolidation should be dull to percussion.

4.009 In a patient with a pleural effusion, which of the following signs would you NOT expect to find?
 A. wheezes would be heard over involved area
 B. breath sounds would be decreased over involved area
 C. percussion would be dull or flat over involved side
 D. tactile fremitus would be decreased over involved area

A is correct.
Adventitious sounds are not present, unless there is underlying disease of the lung.

4.010 Which of the following statements is true about a friction rub?
 A. a friction rub will usually be heard during inspiration and expiration
 B. friction rubs may frequently be heard in normal patients
 C. friction rubs are generally caused by narrowing of the airways
 D. friction rubs are heard in epiglottis

A is correct.
Representing the impaired sliding of the pleura, rubs are usually heard in both inspiration and expiration, though occasionally only in inspiration.

4.011 Regular, cyclically increasing and decreasing respirations alternating with periods of apnea BEST describe what respiratory pattern?
 A. Kussmaul's respirations
 B. Biot's breathing
 C. Cheyne-Stokes respirations
 D. ataxic breathing

C is correct.
May be normal in sleeping children or elderly. Pathological causes include heart failure, uremia, and drugs, among others.

4.012 Clubbing of the nails is present if the angle between the nail and its bed is _____ and the base feels _____.
    A. increased; firm
    B. decreased; firm
    C. increased; spongy
    D. decreased; spongy

C is correct.
Normal angle is about 160¡; with clubbing, the angle increases to greater than 180¡, and the nail bed becomes spongy to compression.

4.013 Physical signs of respiratory distress include all of the following EXCEPT:
    A. flaring nares
    B. use of sternocleidomastoid muscles
    C. pursed lips
    D. leaning forward with arms braced
    E. preference for lying flat

E is correct.
Lying flat causes the abdominal contents to elevate the diaphragms and would increase dyspnea in a patient in respiratory distress. (Remember Thanksgiving dinner?)

4.014 Cyanosis in an adult:
    A. results from minimal desaturation of hemoglobin
    B. results from the formation of small quantities of carboxyhemoglobin
    C. represents significant desaturation of hemoglobin
    D. represents high percentages of carboxyhemoglobin

C is correct.
Kids can readily (and often do) hold their breath till they are "blue in the face" to manipulate Mom. On the other hand, adults who are cyanotic are significantly hypoxemic.

4.015 A patient presents with respiratory distress after striking his chest on the steering wheel in a motor vehicle accident. On exam, you note diminished breath sounds on the right, with hyperresonance on the right and tracheal deviation to the left. This suggests:
    A. simple pneumothorax on the right
    B. tension pneumothorax on the right
    C. tension pneumothorax on the left
    D. hemothorax on the right

B is correct.
Decreased BS tell us the right side is the affected side. Simple pneumo would cause tracheal deviation toward the affected side and more or less symmetric percussion sounds. Tension pneumo is consistent with the description, with the hyperresonant percussion on the affected side. Hemothorax would cause dullness on the affected side.

4.016 A patient presents with respiratory distress after striking his chest on the steering wheel in an MVA. On exam, you note diminished breath sounds on the right, with hyperresonance on the right and tracheal deviation to the left. The patient also exhibits JVD, which:
    A. supports the diagnosis of simple pneumothorax but may also result from cardiac tamponade
    B. supports the diagnosis of tension pneumothorax
    C. supports the diagnosis of tension pneumothorax but may also result from cardiac tamponade
    D. may only result from cardiac tamponade in this patient

C is correct.
After blunt chest trauma, either condition may exist and both can have associated JVD.

4.017 Which characteristic of sputum listed is MOST indicative of infection?
    A. quantity
    B. viscosity
    C. color
    D. source

C is correct.
Sputum quantity can vary for noninfectious reasons (like allergy/asthma). Viscosity is affected by hydration and other factors. Mucus may arise in nasal passages or the airways due to allergens, irritants, and other stimuli.

4.018 Probably the MOST important contributory factor to the development of chronic obstructive pulmonary disease is:
  A. environmental pollution
  B. work exposure to coal dust
  C. work exposure to asbestos
  D. tobacco smoking

D is correct.
While exposure to other irritants, such as air pollution and work exposures, may contribute to COPD, their contribution pales (no pun intended) when compared with the effects of smoking. Asbestos exposure is specifically a risk factor for mesothelioma, and coal dust exposure causes "black lung disease."

4.019 Symptomatic COPD is:
  A. often irreversible
  B. always curable
  C. a minor cause of total disability
  D. never reversible
  E. rarely disabling

D is correct.
COPD is a major cause of disability in the U.S. While its effects are manageable in many patients, it is typically irreversible and progressive.

4.020 The spectrum of diseases called COPD shares what common pathology?
  A. chronic slowing of the expiratory flow rate
  B. chronic inflammation of the airways
  C. chronic infection of the small airways
  D. excess mucus production of high viscosity
  E. loss of intra-alveolar septa and surface area for gas exchange

A is correct.
While all the other components may exist in one or another form of COPD at times, the final common pathology is the decreased expiratory flow rate.

4.021 The earliest manifestation of COPD seems to be:
  A. a decrease in small airway resistance
  B. an increase in small airway resistance
  C. a decrease in large airway resistance
  D. an increase in large airway resistance
  E. decreases in both large and small airway resistance

B is correct.
The disease affects small airways first, resulting in an increase in resistance to airflow.

4.022 Clinical presentation of a patient with COPD includes:
  A. dyspnea
  B. cough
  C. sputum production
  D. wheezing
  E. any combination of the above

E is correct.
While all need not be present in any one patient at any one time, these are the major clinical manifestations of COPD.

4.023 The single MOST important therapeutic intervention for patients with newly diagnosed COPD is:
  A. influenza and pneumococcal vaccines
  B. bronchodilators
  C. smoking cessation
  D. theophylline
  E. corticosteroids
  F. anticholinergics

C is correct.
Smoking cessation may arrest or delay progression of the disease and significantly improve pulmonary function.

4.024 Known stimuli for asthma include:
  A. allergens, exercise, respiratory infection, heat
  B. heat, exercise, respiratory infection, irritants
  C. allergens, heat, respiratory infection, irritants
  D. allergens, exercise, heat, irritants
  E. allergens, exercise, respiratory infection, irritants

E is correct.
All of these may precipitate bronchospasm in an asthmatic. Exercise on cold, dry days has been shown to trigger asthma.

4.025 The two MOST common etiologies of hemoptysis are:
   A. bronchogenic carcinoma and pneumonia
   B. chronic bronchitis and bronchiectasis
   C. tuberculosis and vascular lesions
   D. tuberculosis and excessive anticoagulant therapy
   E. acute and chronic bronchitis

E is correct.
While the other entities listed all cause hemoptysis, acute and chronic bronchitis are the most common etiologies.

4.026 Initial diagnostic studies for hemoptysis include:
   A. chest x-ray
   B. chest CT
   C. sputum cytology
   D. bronchoscopy
   E. bleeding studies

A is correct.
Chest x-ray, sputum Gram stain (if purulent), sputum acid-fast stain (and PPD skin test if needed) constitute initial evaluation. Other exams listed may be entertained as follow-up studies, if indicated by the initial workup.

4.027 Bronchoscopy is NOT indicated in a patient with hemoptysis:
   A. if the diagnosis is still in doubt after the initial workup
   B. who has massive hemoptysis and is being considered for surgery
   C. who quit smoking
   D. routinely

D is correct.
Routine bronchoscopy is not done, as the yield is very low in patients at low risk for having tumors.

4.028 In a patient with fever and a cough, sputum Gram stain shows "polys" and lancet-shaped gram-positive cocci in pairs. The MOST likely organism listed is:
   A. *Haemophilus influenzae* (−)
   B. *Neisseria meningitidis* (−)
   C. *Streptococcus pneumoniae* (+)
   D. *Staphylococcus aureus* (+)
   E. *Legionella pneumophila* (−)

C is correct.
The organisms given in A, B and E are gram-negative rods, and staphylococci appear rounder and in grape-like clusters.

4.029 Intra-alveolar exudation in pneumonia results in:
   A. bronchiectasis
   B. consolidation
   C. atelectasis
   D. necrosis
   E. edema

B is correct.
The hallmark of bacterial pneumonia is the consolidation of a lobar segment of lung due to suppurative exudates in the alveoli.

4.030 Cold agglutinins in a patient with clinical pneumonia suggest:
   A. *H. influenzae*
   B. *Mycobacterium tuberculosis*
   C. *S. pneumoniae*
   D. *Mycoplasma*
   E. *Legionella*

D is correct.
Cold agglutinins are specific for mycoplasmal pneumonia, a common finding in young adults in closed settings such as military barracks or schools.

4.031 A 20-year-old nonsmoking woman presents, complaining of nonproductive cough, low-grade fever, and chest tightness for 4 days. Symptoms have increased gradually and follow a 7-day course of malaise, rhinorrhea, and sinus pressure. Self-care with OTC medications has limited but not alleviated the symptoms. PMH/FMH are noncontributory. The MOST likely cause of the problem is:
   A. post-URI bronchospasm
   B. COPD
   C. pneumonia
   D. reactive airways disease
   E. acute bronchitis

E is correct.
This is a typical presentation of acute bronchitis. The negative PMH mitigates against any chronic condition such as COPD or asthma (reactive airways disease). Post-URI bronchospasm would not account for the fever. Pneumonia is possible but less likely than bronchitis and would need to be ruled out on exam.

4.032 On physical exam of this patient, which finding is would be MOST diagnostic of bronchitis:
   A. clear rhinorrhea
   B. retracted tympanic membranes
   C. lack of sinus tenderness
   D. diffuse wheezes
   E. pharyngeal erythema

D is correct.
Wheezes are commonly heard in patients with acute bronchitis. The other findings suggest the URI prodrome described by the patient.

4.033 Peak flow measurement in this patient is 75% of expected; the BEST immediate treatment is:
   A. theophylline
   B. β_1-agonists
   C. β_2-agonists
   D. steroids
   E. antibiotics

C is correct.
Short-term β_2-agonist therapy is indicated for symptomatic relief in this patient. Steroids should be avoided in patients with infections. Empirical antibiotic therapy will have no immediate effect on the patient's respiratory status.

4.034 Empirical antibiotic treatment in this patient may consist of:
   A. erythromycin
   B. amoxicillin
   C. trimethoprim/sulfamethoxazole
   D. tetracycline
   E. any of the above

E is correct.
All of these agents have been used successfully for empirical therapy of acute bronchitis (probably because many cases are viral in origin and self-limited anyway).

4.035 Chest x-ray in this patient reveals no infiltrates; therefore, the patient MOST likely has:
   A. acute bronchitis
   B. early pneumonia
   C. atypical pneumonia syndrome
   D. pneumonia
   E. *Klebsiella* pneumonia

A is correct.
Normal CXR in this patient continues to support the working diagnosis of acute bronchitis. It should be noted, however, that this does not rule out pneumonia, as the CXR findings can lag behind the clinical course of pneumonia.

4.036 Cough suppression in this patient should be:
   A. as near total as possible to maximize patient comfort
   B. as needed to a maximum of q1 hour
   C. daytime use only
   D. nighttime use only to allow sleep
   E. totally avoided

D is correct.
Coughing to clear secretions in the daytime should be encouraged. Sleep-disturbing cough interferes with the body's ability to clear the infection and should be suppressed.

4.037 Fluid intake in this patient should be:
  A. minimized
  B. ad lib but discouraged
  C. ad lib
  D. at least 200 cc/day
  E. at least 2000 cc/day

E is correct.
Adequate hydration is essential to clearing respiratory secretions.

4.038 Expectorants have:
  A. no role in acute bronchitis
  B. no role in acute pneumonia
  C. some sputum-loosening effects
  D. clearly demonstrated effect on clinical outcome
  E. become contraindicated in lower respiratory tract diseases

C is correct.
Expectorants have been shown to loosen secretions; their use has not been clearly demonstrated to have an effect on clinical outcome.

4.039 The primary pathogenesis of asthma is:
  A. allergy-mediated bronchospasm
  B. chronic inflammation
  C. excess secretion of viscid mucus
  D. irritant-mediated bronchospasm

B is correct.
While all of these have some role in asthma, chronic inflammation seems to be primary and justifies the emphasis on anti-inflammatory agents in the management of the disease.

4.040 A 6-year-old boy is brought to the ER, having an "asthma attack." The BEST way to assess his oxygenation is by:
  A. clinical signs of respiratory distress
  B. peak flow measurements
  C. pulse oximetry
  D. arterial blood gases
  E. vital signs

C is correct.
The least invasive, most direct measure of oxygenation available is the pulse oximeter. Vital signs and clinical assessment are qualitative at best for assessing oxygenation. ABGs are invasive, painful, and slow. Peak flow measurement indicates ventilation not oxygenation, and the correlation between them varies with individuals.

4.041 The BEST initial medication for this patient is:
  A. cromolyn
  B. β-agonist
  C. anticholinergic
  D. MAST cell stabilizing agent
  E. steroids

B is correct.
β-agonists are the mainstay of therapy to relieve *acute* bronchospasm.

4.042 The BEST route of administration listed is:
  A. oral
  B. PR
  C. nebulized with oxygen
  D. nebulized with air
  E. SQ

C is correct.
Oxygen is preferred over air in this patient to relieve hypoxemia and prevent sudden drops in P_{AO_2} caused by blood return from shunt fractions in the lung.

4.043 Mom states that she gave him additional nebulized doses of his medicine—cromolyn (Intal®)—this AM without relief. This is likely due to:
  A. severity of attack
  B. difficulty administering the medication while wheezing
  C. inappropriate route of administration
  D. wrong medicine
  E. reaching maximum effect of the drug with the initial dose

D is correct.
Cromolyn is a MAST cell stabilizing agent useful for preventing the development of allergy-mediated symptoms and has no role in the relief of acute symptoms.

4.044 Which of the following is NOT suggestive of extrinsic asthma in this patient?
  A. eczema
  B. food allergies
  C. environmental allergies
  D. URI triggers
  E. elevated IgE

D is correct.
URI triggers asthmatic complaints in most patients with reactive airways.

4.045 The MOST important information from ABGs in the acute asthmatic is:
  A. O_2 saturation
  B. pO_2
  C. pCO_2
  D. HCO_3
  E. base excess

C is correct.
If you have done ABGs, the pCO_2 is the best indicator of ventilation. Hopefully, it will be decreased, indicating hyperventilation in response to hypoxemia. As the attack progresses, it rises through normal to elevated. Therefore, if it is normal, where are we?

4.046 The MOST sensitive test for tuberculosis is:
  A. chest x-ray
  B. sputum for AFB
  C. sputum culture
  D. bronchoscopy
  E. PPD skin test

E is correct.
In immunocompetent patients!

4.047 Which statement is FALSE about BCG?
  A. it is not generally used in the U.S.
  B. it is a vaccine against TB
  C. it is recommended for household contacts of people with +PPD
  D. it is not given to persons with +PPD.

C is correct.
Household contacts of converters are not routinely treated, unless active pulmonary disease is demonstrated.

4.048 A 28-year-old PA student presents to your office for a physical before entering the clinical year. He is asymptomatic and has a normal PE. There is no history of TB exposure known, but he worked as a nurse in a corrections facility. His last PPD was negative 14 months ago when he left the facility. At this time, you should:
  A. perform only a TB tine screening
  B. perform a 5-unit intradermal PPD
  C. perform a TB tine and a CXR
  D. perform a CXR alone
  E. obtain sputum for AFB

B is correct.
In asymptomatic individuals, the intradermal PPD is the best way to assess exposure.

4.049 If you elect to do an intradermal PPD, it should be read:
  A. by the patient at 24 hours
  B. by the provider at 24 hours
  C. by the patient at 48–72 hours
  D. by the provider at 48–72 hours
  E. by the provider in 1 week to check for booster effect

D is correct.
Although some places rely on patient reports.

4.050 The patient returns to the office in 48 hours, complaining of erythema 50 mm in diameter around the test site:
    A. this is a positive reaction
    B. this is a positive reaction if documented by the provider
    C. this is a positive reaction only if induration of at least 10 mm is also found
    D. this is a positive reaction only if no induration is found
    E. this is a negative reaction if more than 10 mm of induration is associated with it

C is correct.
The criteria for positive PPD are based on the presence and degree of induration—not erythema.

4.051 You conclude the patient has a positive PPD. Further studies for TB in this patient:
    A. are not needed
    B. should include CXR
    C. should include CXR and sputum for AFB
    D. should include CXR, sputum culture and AFB
    E. should include sputum culture and AFB

B is correct.
CXR is necessary to identify active pulmonary disease.

4.052 This patient should be treated:
    A. only if PPD, CXR, and AFB are positive
    B. only if CXR and PPD are positive
    C. only if CXR is positive
    D. if PPD is positive
    E. only if all studies (PPD, CXR, AFB, and culture) confirm active disease

D is correct.
PPD documents exposure that requires treatment to prevent the development of active disease, even in asymptomatic patients with a normal CXR.

4.053 The oxygen device of choice for low percentages of inspired oxygen is:
    A. nasal cannula
    B. simple face mask
    C. bag-valve mask
    D. non-rebreather mask
    E. partial rebreather mask

A is correct.
Nasal cannulas are generally tolerated better than face masks.

4.054 The oxygen device of choice for maximum percentages of inspired oxygen in conscious patients is:
    A. nasal cannula
    B. simple face mask
    C. Venturi mask
    D. non-rebreather mask
    E. partial rebreather mask

D is correct.
The non-rebreather mask provides the highest percentage of inspired oxygen in patients who are breathing adequately on their own.

4.055 FIO_2 of room air is:
    A. 11%
    B. 21%
    C. 31%
    D. 41%
    E. 51%

B is correct.
Of which we utilize 3%, leaving 18% for mouth to mask if needed (remember your CPR?).

4.056 Hazards of oxygen therapy in adults include all of the following EXCEPT:
 A. oxygen-induced hypoventilation
 B. absorption atelectasis
 C. O₂ toxicity
 D. retrolental fibroplasia

D is correct.
Retrolental fibroplasia is a condition affecting infants.

4.057 Hazards of metered-dose inhalers may include all of the following EXCEPT:
 A. bronchospasm
 B. medication side effects
 C. overdose
 D. oral thrush
 E. esophageal candidiasis

E is correct.
Oral thrush with inhaled steroids. Esophageal candidiasis should suggest immune compromise rather than use of a steroid MDI.

4.058 Chest physical therapy (CPT) is BEST defined as:
 A. gravity-assisted bronchial drainage aided by percussion of the chest wall
 B. a pneumatic pulsation device producing chest compression
 C. therapy that uses the patient's own muscular efforts to accomplish hyperinflation
 D. exhaling with pursed lips in a slow manner
 E. placing hand over affected lung field and applying pressure during the expiratory phase

A is correct.
Useful in patients who have difficulty clearing secretions.

4.059 The BEST way to improve delivery from a metered-dose inhaler is to have the patient:
 A. sit while using the device
 B. hold breath for 5 seconds before inhaling
 C. breath in as rapidly as possible while releasing the medication
 D. use a spacer device

D is correct.
Proper training in use of the MDI is essential, but spacers make it much easier and more effective.

4.060 A useful technique for assessing the quantity of medication in a MDI is to:
 A. shake it and see how it sounds
 B. spray it into the air and see how far the mist goes
 C. weigh it on an accurate pan balance
 D. see how high it floats in water

D is correct.
You can also weigh it, but most law-abiding patients will not have access to an accurate pan balance.

TEST PLAN FOR SECTION 4: RESPIRATORY SYSTEM

Tasks/areas assessed	Hx and PE	Dx studies	Diagnosis	Prognosis	Health maintenance	Management		Applying scientific concepts
						Clinical intervention	Clinical therapeutics	
				question numbers				
Total questions = 60	13	9	8	4	6	6	8	6
Diseases/disorders								
Acute bronchitis	6		31,32	35		36,37	33,34,38	
Acute bronchiolitis								
Croup								
Influenza								
Pneumonia	8	28,30	2,3					29
Asthma	7	40,45			57,59,60		41–43	24,39,44
Chronic airway obstruction								
Chronic bronchitis	25	26						
Obstructive chronic bronchitis	22		21	19	18	23,58		20
Other emphysema	17							
Pneumoconiosis due to silica/asbestos								
Neoplasms	12	27		1				
Pleural effusion	9							
Pleurisy, no effusion	10							
Pneumothorax	4,5		15,16					
Pulmonary embolism/infection								
Pulmonary tuberculosis	11,13	46,49,50	51		47,48		52	
Respiratory distress syndrome				14		53,54	56	55
Sarcoidosis								

SECTION 5: CIRCULATORY SYSTEM

5.001 A normal S_1 is:
- A. heard best with diaphragm, at the base
- B. heard best with bell, at the apex
- C. heard best with diaphragm, at the apex
- D. heard best with bell, at the base

C is correct.

S_1 represents closure of the atrioventricular (AV) valves, with the left-sided mitral valve component loudest—therefore heard best over the apex. Because it is a higher-pitched sound, it will be heard better with the diaphragm of the stethoscope.

5.002 A normal S_2 is:
- A. heard best with diaphragm, at the base
- B. heard best with bell, at the apex
- C. heard best with diaphragm, at the apex
- D. heard best with bell, at the base

A is correct.

S_2 represents closure of the semilunar valves, with the left-sided aortic valve component loudest—therefore heard best over the base. Because it is a higher-pitched sound, it will be heard better with the diaphragm of the stethoscope.

5.003 A normal S_3 is:
- A. relatively high pitched, heard best at the base
- B. relatively low pitched, heard best at the base
- C. relatively high pitched, heard best at the apex
- D. relatively low pitched, heard best at the apex
- E. does not occur

D is correct.
May be pathological or normal.

S_4 = atrial kick

5.004 A murmur heard from S_1 through to the next S_1 at a constant pitch and volume is:
- A. pansystolic, plateau murmur
- B. continuous, plateau murmur
- C. continuous, decrescendo murmur
- D. continuous, diamond-shaped murmur
- E. pansystolic, decrescendo murmur

B is correct.

5.005 Extra sounds in systole include:
- A. ejection sounds, split S_1, clicks
- B. ejection sounds, split S_1, opening snap
- C. ejection sounds, opening snap, clicks
- D. split S_1, opening snap, clicks
- E. split S_1, opening snap, S_4

A is correct.
Opening snap of mitral stenosis and the atrial sound (S_4) are heard in diastole.

5.006 S_1-S_2-S_3-S_4 represents:
- A. a summation gallop associated with tachycardia
- B. a summation gallop associated with heart failure
- C. tachycardia when beats are too close together to identify S_1
- D. multiple extra-high-pitched sounds in systole (mitral valve prolapse)

B is correct.
At rapid rates, the S_3 and S_4 merge into one loud sound.

5.007 A harsh, rumbling IV/VI holosystolic, decrescendo murmur heard best at the right second intercostal space is MOST likely:
  A. aortic stenosis
  B. aortic insufficiency
  C. mitral stenosis
  D. tricuspid stenosis

A is correct.
AI, mitral stenosis, and tricuspid stenosis would all result in diastolic murmurs.

5.008 In a patient with an AV junctional rhythm, the stimulus for the heart to contract may be conducted backward (retrograde) from the AV node to the atrium. Which represents the correct sequence for retrograde conduction?
  A. AV node, internodal pathways, SA node
  B. AV node, bundle of His, SA node
  C. AV node, internodal pathways, bundle of His
  D. AV node, bundle of His, L/R bundle branches, Purkinje fibers

A is correct.

5.009 The property of automaticity:
  A. is unique to cardiac and smooth muscle
  B. allows only specialized cells in the myocardium to function as a potential pacemaker
  C. provides for contraction without electrical stimulation
  D. is also found in striated muscle
  E. allows the heart to beat only when autonomic nervous system is functional

C is correct.
Unique to cardiac muscle, this is why that frog heart continues to beat in the Petri dish.

5.010 The intrinsic firing rate of the AV node is:
  A. 100–120
  B. 60–100
  C. 40–60
  D. <40

C is correct.
Nodal rhythms are slower than sinus or atrial, but faster than those of ventricular origin.

5.011 The time during which an impulse, no matter how strong, cannot stimulate a premature contraction is the:
  A. absolute refractory period
  B. depolarization phase
  C. relative refractory period
  D. repolarization phase
  E. isoelectric phase

A is correct.
During the relative refractory period, strong impulses can trigger contractions and fibrillation may result.

5.012 The time from the beginning of the P wave to the first deflection of the QRS is:
  A. P–P interval
  B. QRS interval
  C. ST segment
  D. R–R interval
  E. P–R interval

E is correct.
Or PRI for short. It represents conduction of the stimulus from the SA node through the AV node and to the ventricles.

5.013 The normal PRI is ___ sec.
  A. <0.12
  B. <0.10
  C. 0.12–0.20
  D. 0.05–0.20
  E. 0.08–0.15

C is correct.
Short PRIs suggest abnormal accessory conduction, as in Wolff-Parkinson-White syndrome, and prolonged PRI is at least first-degree AV block.

5.014 One small square on the monitor paper represents ___ sec.
  A. 0.10
  B. 0.02
  C. 0.03
  D. 0.04
  E. 0.20

D is correct.
Therefore, our PRI is normally 3–5 small squares.

5.015 Upright P waves in lead II:
  A. are normal
  B. are retrograde
  C. indicate ectopic pacemaker
  D. may indicate junctional pacemaker
  E. may indicate ventricular pacemaker

A is correct.
The positive end of the lead II axis is in the direction of the current flow; therefore, the deflection is upward.

5.016 A normal QRS is less than ___ sec.
  A. 0.05
  B. 0.12
  C. 0.18
  D. 0.20
  E. 0.25

B is correct.
Or three small boxes.

5.017 Failure of the ST segment to return to the isoelectric line may be indicative of:
  A. ischemia
  B. hyperkalemia
  C. hypokalemia
  D. bundle branch block
  E. hypertrophy

A is correct.
Potassium level is reflected on the ECG by the height of the T wave. Bundle branch block affects the timing of the QRS complex and hypertrophy the magnitude of the ECG signals.

5.018 The pacemaker site for sinus arrhythmia is:
  A. SA node
  B. atrial ectopic
  C. AV node
  D. AV junction
  E. ventricular

A is correct.
A misnomer, as arrhythmia is the absence of a rhythm. Sinus arrhythmia is the physiologic variation in the heart rate (and therefore the P–P intervals) with respiration.

5.019 The QRS of a PAC is:
  A. usually normal
  B. wide and bizarre
  C. biphasic
  D. always >0.15
  E. absent

A is correct.
An ectopic source in the atria produces the impulse, but since it follows the normal conduction via the AV node to the ventricles, it registers with a "normal" QRS. That is one that looks like those of a sinus beat in this patient.

5.020 Irregularly irregular pulse of 100, absent P wave, and normal QRS BEST describe:
  A. atrial tachycardia
  B. atrial fibrillation
  C. atrial flutter
  D. PSVT
  E. SVT

B is correct.
Irregularly irregular pulses are almost always atrial fib.

5.021 Regular R–R and P–P intervals but no relationship between P waves and QRS's:
    A. 1° AV Block
    B. 2° AV block, type I
    C. 2° AV block, type II
    D. 3° AV block
    E. atrial fib

D is correct.
In lower grades of block, some association is maintained between the P's and the QRS's. In atrial fib P's and therefore P–P intervals cannot be identified.

5.022 An inferior wall myocardial infarction will have significant (abnormal) Q waves in:
    A. V_1 to V_3
    B. aVR and aVL
    C. II, III, and AVF
    D. V_4 to V_6

C is correct.
Findings in these leads localize to the inferior wall of the heart.

Questions 5.023–5.029 refer to ECG #1 (next page).
5.023 The rate in this ECG is about ___ beats/min.
    A. 150
    B. 125
    C. 75
    D. 60
    E. 50

D is correct.
Count from a complex that falls on the 0.20-sec marks. Count 300-150-100-75-60 for each 0.20-sec mark, noting that the next beat falls closest to the fifth mark "60."

5.024 The rhythm in this ECG is BEST described as:
    A. sinus
    B. sinus bradycardia
    C. sinus bradycardia with 1° AV block
    D. tachycardia
    E. junctional

C is correct.
The rate is just slightly <60/min, and the PRI is >0.20 sec.

5.025 The axis for this ECG is:
    A. RAD about 180°
    B. RAD about 150°
    C. normal about 0°
    D. LAD about –30°
    E. LAD about 90°

C is correct.
Using beats 1–3 as the "normals," lead I is up, so the axis is to the left. Lead aVF is also up, so the axis is left and down. With aVF, also the most isoelectric, the axis is in the left lower quadrant at right angles to aVF. Therefore, normal at 0°.

5.026 This ECG suggests hypertrophy of which part of the heart?
    A. RA
    B. RV
    C. LA
    D. LV
    E. none

C is correct.
P in lead I is ≥0.11 sec (barely), with terminal negative deflection of the P in V_1. This suggests left atrial hypertrophy.

5.027 Both left and right bundle branch blocks are ruled out by the absence of:
    A. QRS >0.12
    B. RSR' in V_1
    C. ST depressions
    D. T-wave inversions in I, aVL, V_5, V_6
    E. no one criterion can rule out both left and right BBB

A is correct.
QRS must be >0.12 sec to have either a left or right BBB. The other criteria apply to RBBB (B) and LBBB (C,D).

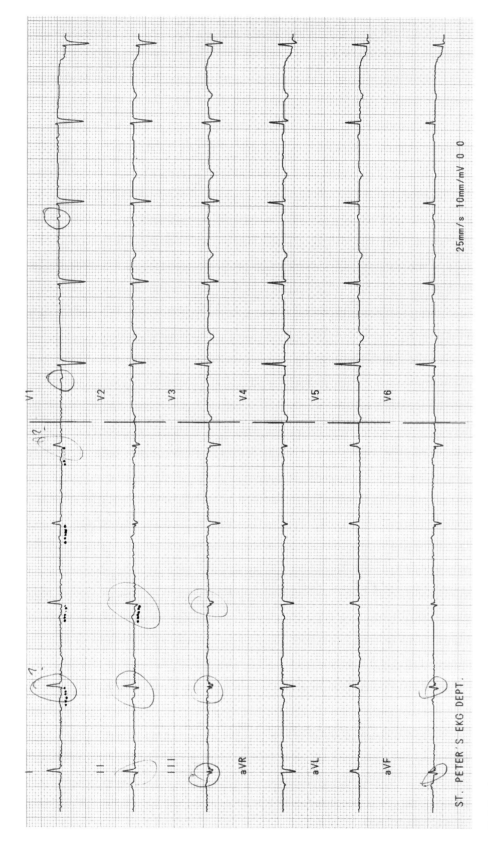

25mm/s 10mm/mV 0 0

ST. PETER'S EKG DEPT.

ECG #I

5.028 Which leads of this ECG show significant Q waves?
A. I, V_2–V_4
B. I, aVL, V_5–V_6
C. II, III
D. III, aVR, V_1
E. none of them

C is correct.
Q's $\geq$0.04 mm or $\geq$25% of R wave appear in II and III and are significant.

5.029 These findings are consistent with:
A. anterior MI
B. anterolateral MI
C. inferior MI
D. acute anterior wall MI only
E. normal ECG

C is correct.
Q's in II, III, and aVF are consistent with inferior wall MI. Age of the infarct cannot be determined.

Questions 5.030–5.036 refer to ECG #2 (next page).
5.030 The rate in this ECG is about ___ beats/min.
A. 150
B. 100
C. 75
D. 60
E. 50

C is correct.
Count from a complex that falls on the 0.20-sec marks. Count 300-150-100-75 for each 0.20-sec mark, noting that the next beat falls closest to the fourth mark "75."

5.031 The rhythm in this ECG is BEST described as:
A. sinus
B. sinus tachycardia
C. sinus bradycardia
D. sinus bradycardia with PAC
E. sinus with PVC

A is correct.
This is a RSR' at about 75/min.

5.032 The axis for this ECG is:
A. RAD about 180°
B. RAD about 120°
C. normal about 90°
D. LAD about –30°
E. LAD about –90°

C is correct.
Lead I is positive, indicating that the axis points to the patient's left. Lead aVF is positive, so the axis is down (and left) between 0° and 90°. Lead I is the most isoelectric of the limb leads, and a perpendicular to it in the left lower quadrant would fall at 90°.

5.033 This ECG suggests hypertrophy of which part of the heart?
A. RA
B. RV
C. LA
D. LV
E. none

C is correct.
None of the criteria for hypertrophy is met.

5.034 Which lead shows an RSR'?
A. I
B. aVR
C. V_1
D. V_3
E. none of the leads

E is correct.
RSR' is a double upward deflection in the QRS and may resemble rabbit ears.

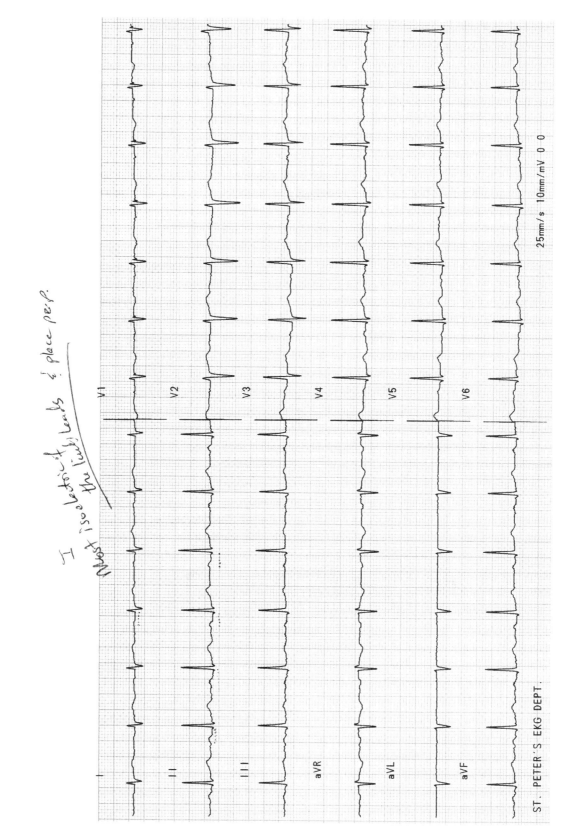

I isoelectric it
the limb leads ¿ place PERP.
Most isoelectric it

V1
V2
V3
V4
V5
V6

I
II
III
aVR
aVL
aVF

25mm/s 10mm/mV 0 0

ST. PETER'S EKG DEPT.

ECG #2

5.035 Which lead of this ECG shows significant Q's?
   A. I
   B. III
   C. aVR
   D. V$_1$
   E. none of the leads

E is correct.
Q's in aVR are ignored. No other Q's ≥0.04 mm or ≥25% R wave appear.

5.036 These findings are consistent with:
   A. anterior MI
   B. anterolateral MI
   C. inferior MI
   D. acute anterior wall MI only
   E. normal ECG

E is correct.
This ECG is normal.

5.037 Causes of physiological murmurs include all of the following EXCEPT:
   A. exercise
   B. asymmetric septal hypertrophy
   C. fever
   D. pregnancy
   E. anemia

B is correct.
Asymmetric septal hypertrophy is the pathology of IHSS and cannot produce a "physiologic" murmur.

5.038 A late systolic murmur introduced by a mid-systolic click signifies:
   A. a small ventricular septal defect
   B. mitral insufficiency
   C. tricuspid insufficiency
   D. mitral valve prolapse
   E. none of the above

D is correct.
This "click-murmur syndrome" is associated with symptoms in some patients.

5.039 The MOST typical murmur heard with rheumatic heart disease is:
   A. mitral valve prolapse
   B. rupture of the chordae tendineae
   C. mitral insufficiency with hemodynamically significant regurgitation
   D. aortic stenosis
   E. none of the above

C is correct.
As "typical" as can be given, how uncommon RHD has become!

5.040 On auscultation of the heart in a new patient, you hear a diastolic murmur. This:
   A. is a normal variant
   B. may be pathological but is a likely normal variant
   C. may be a normal variant, but is likely pathological
   D. is always pathological

D is correct.
Diastolic murmurs are always pathological.

5.041 This murmur may be:
   A. AS, PS, MR, TR
   B. AR, PR, MS, TS
   C. AR, PR, MR, TR
   D. AS, PS, MS, TS

B is correct.
Diastolic (valvular) murmurs represent narrowing of AV valves (M/TS) or regurgitation of semilunar valves (A/PR).

5.042 Which of the following murmurs are all heard during diastole?
   A. aortic stenosis, mitral stenosis, patent ductus arteriosus
   B. aortic regurgitation, mitral regurgitation, patent ductus arteriosus
   C. aortic regurgitation, mitral stenosis, patent ductus arteriosus
   D. aortic stenosis, mitral stenosis, ventricular septal defect
   E. aortic regurgitation, mitral regurgitation, ventricular septal defect

C is correct.
The murmurs of AR and MS are heard in diastole as blood flows backward across the incompetent aortic valve (AR) or forward through the narrowed mitral valve (MS). PDA causes a continuous murmur with components in both systole and diastole as blood flows through the open pathway provided by the ductus.

5.043 Which of the following is FALSE concerning supraventricular tachycardias?
   A. they can occur in normal hearts
   B. they can occur with Wolff-Parkinson-White syndrome
   C. they may be precipitated by caffeine
   D. resolution is typically abrupt
   E. vagal maneuvers are not useful in their treatment

E is correct.
Vagal maneuvers like the Valsalva maneuver or carotid sinus massage may be used to "break" SVTs.

5.044 In patients with atrial fibrillation, it is important to keep the rate:
   A. under 85 at rest
   B. under 120 at rest
   C. under 110 with mild exercise
   D. under 140 with mild exercise
   E. A and C

E is correct.
Too rapid a ventricular response may impair cardiac output by decreasing filling time, decrease coronary perfusion, and increase the myocardial oxygen demand.

5.045 An 18-year-old female presents, complaining of palpitations occurring in episodes that come on and resolve spontaneously and gradually. She states that her radial pulse is regular and rapid when they occur (she is tennis player and was taught to check pulse in training). The LEAST likely cause listed is:
   A. exertion
   B. emotion
   C. medications
   D. stimulants
   E. pheochromocytoma

E is correct.
Remember: "When you hear hoof beats, think horses, not zebras." Any of these might be the cause, but pheo is rare (a zebra). All of the others are common (horses).

5.046 Associated symptoms that, if present in this patient, would be suggestive of heart disease include:
   A. dyspnea, chest pain, syncope
   B. chest tightness, air hunger at rest
   C. breast tenderness, nausea, missed menses
   D. malaise, sore throat, chest congestion

A is correct.
B suggests respiratory causes, C pregnancy, and D viral infection.

5.047 Which of the following are all associated with palpitations?
- A. OTC cold remedies, theophylline, tricyclic antidepressants, digitalis, anticholinergics
- B. acetaminophen, theophylline, tricyclic antidepressants, digitalis, anticholinergics
- C. OTC cold remedies, tricyclic antidepressants, digitalis, NSAIDs
- D. OTC cold remedies, theophylline, digitalis, anticholinergics, antibiotics

A is correct.
Although I follow the "any symptom, any patient, any drug, any time" rule of side effects, NSAIDs, antibiotics (alone), and acetaminophen are not commonly associated with palpitations.

5.048 The patient's PMH is significant for asthma and IDDM; you suggest that her symptoms may result from:
- A. hyperglycemia secondary to insulin in excess of food
- B. hyperglycemia due to prolonged exercise
- C. hypoglycemia due to skipped meals
- D. hypoglycemia due to food in excess of insulin

C is correct.
Hypoglycemia is a possible cause of palpitations.

5.049 She advises you that she checked her sugar by glucometer at the time of the last episode of palpitations and it was 105. Presuming the reading was accurate, this:
- A. confirms your suspicion
- B. does not rule out your suspicion but doesn't confirm it either
- C. rules out your suspicion

C is correct.
Hypoglycemia in conjunction with symptoms is required to make the etiological connection. This blood sugar effectively rules this out as the problem.

5.050 The pulse assessment in this patient is BEST done:
- A. apically
- B. at carotid
- C. femorally
- D. radially

A is correct.
Symptomatic extrasystoles may not be strong enough to produce a peripheral pulse, so an apical pulse check is needed in this patient.

5.051 The initial evaluation to reach the diagnosis of essential hypertension should include all of the following EXCEPT:
- A. serial BP determinations
- B. history and PE
- C. electrolytes, BUN, glucose, urinalysis
- D. ECG
- E. 24-hour urine for metanephrine

E is correct.
This is used to diagnose pheochromocytoma.

5.052 β-Blockers should be avoided in what two specific groups of patients?
- A. asthmatics and patients with migraines
- B. hypertensives and women
- C. black men and diabetics
- D. diabetics and asthmatics
- E. elderly men and white women

D is correct.
Beta-blockade may produce bronchospasm in asthmatics and mask hypoglycemic symptoms in diabetics.

5.053 The number one and number two MOST common causes of hypertension (in order) are:
   A. #1 renal, #2 idiopathic
   B. #1 idiopathic, #2 aldosteronism
   C. #1 renal, #2 pheochromocytoma
   D. #1 Cushing's, #2 oral contraceptives
   E. #1 idiopathic, #2 renal

E is correct.
The vast majority of all hypertension is idiopathic (essential or primary), and the leading cause of secondary hypertension is renal disease.

5.054 Most patients with hypertension:
   A. are asymptomatic
   B. have mild symptoms like headache
   C. have syncopal episodes
   D. have chest pain when their BP is elevated

A is correct.
In rare patients, markedly elevated BP may produce symptoms.

5.055 Measurement error for improperly fit cuffs is:
   A. false-low reading if cuff is too large or too small
   B. false-low if cuff too large, false-high if cuff too small
   C. false-low if cuff too small, false-high if cuff too large
   D. false-high if cuff too small or too large

B is correct.
A properly fit cuff is mandatory for accurate BP determinations.

5.056 Hypertension may be diagnosed:
   A. by any one elevated pressure reading
   B. by any difference of 5 mmHg L/R
   C. by any two readings in 1 day
   D. by multiple determinations

D is correct.
Multiple elevated readings must be documented to reach the diagnosis.

5.057 Factors that decrease patient compliance in treating hypertension include:
   A. QD dosing
   B. low cost of medication
   C. lack of significant side effects
   D. lack of symptoms of the disease

D is correct.
Frequent dosing, expensive medication, and significant side effects will reduce compliance in treating hypertensives. The lack of symptoms before and/or after stopping medication promotes noncompliance.

5.058 Which of the following is MOST significant as a cardiac risk factor?
   A. smoking
   B. hypertension
   C. diabetes
   D. family history of sudden cardiac death
   E. sedentary lifestyle

A is correct.

5.059 Which of the following is NOT a risk factor for coronary artery disease?
   A. male gender
   B. diabetes
   C. aspirin consumption
   D. hypertension
   E. cigarette smoking

C is correct.
Aspirin has a demonstrated cardioprotective effect due to its antiplatelet activity.

5.060 Atherosclerosis:
   A. does not usually begin until age 50
   B. occurs only in the coronary arteries
   C. deposits plaque on the intima of the arteries
   D. deposits plaque on the media of the arteries
   E. deposits plaque on the adventitia of the arteries

C is correct.
The atherosclerotic process has been shown to begin in children and affects all arteries.

intima

5.061 The two areas MOST extensively and severely affected by atherosclerosis are:
    A. coronary arteries and carotid arteries
    B. lower abdominal aorta and coronary arteries
    C. lower abdominal aorta and carotid arteries
    D. carotid arteries and circle of Willis

B is correct.
Although any and all arteries can be affected, these are the areas most affected.

5.062 Complicated atheromatous plaques may:
    A. calcify
    B. discharge emboli
    C. develop superimposed thrombi
    D. A and C
    E. all of the above

E is correct.
Leading to all sorts of bad stuff.

5.063 Routine screening of well adults for hypercholesterolemia/hyperlipidemia should include:
    A. fasting total cholesterol and HDL
    B. nonfasting total cholesterol and HDL
    C. nonfasting total cholesterol
    D. nonfasting total cholesterol and LDL
    E. fasting total cholesterol and LDL

B is correct.
The National Cholesterol Education Program recommends these values for screening purposes.

5.064 Decisions regarding the therapy of hypercholesterolemia are based on:
    A. risk factors, proven CAD
    B. proven CAD and LDL
    C. risk factors, proven CAD, and HDL
    D. risk factors
    E. risk factors, proven CAD, and LDL

E is correct.
In the patient with elevated cholesterol, the presence of risk factors, proven CAD, and LDL levels are used to direct therapy.

5.065 Which of the following would have no cholesterol?
    A. milk
    B. butter
    C. eggs
    D. organ meats
    E. margarine

E is correct.
Margarine contains no animal fat, therefore no cholesterol.

5.066 Desirable cholesterol levels are less than:
    A. 200 + age
    B. 300
    C. 250
    D. 200

D is correct.
For now. Some say lower is better.

5.067 The initial treatment of hypercholesterolemia is with:
    A. diet
    B. exercise
    C. weight reduction
    D. all of the above

D is correct.
An initial trial of nonpharmacological interventions is reasonable in virtually all patients.

5.068 Which of the following family medical histories is a risk factor for elevated LDL?
  A. MI in both parents at ages 80, 75
  B. sudden death of father at age 50
  C. sudden death of mother at age 70
  D. MI in father at age 67
  E. type II NIDDM in two siblings

B is correct.
Sudden death before age 50 suggests the possibility of acute MI due to hyperlipidemia.

5.069 Which of the following are all drugs used to lower cholesterol levels?
  A. diuretics, nicotinic acid, "statins"
  B. diuretics, Ca^+channel blockers, oral contraceptives
  C. estrogens, nicotinic acid, oral contraceptives
  D. bile acid sequestrants, nicotinic acid, "statins"
  E. bile acid sequestrants, β-blockers, "statins"

D is correct.
Some oral contraceptives may have deleterious affects on lipid profiles.

5.070 Angina may be precipitated by:
  A. exertion
  B. eating a large meal
  C. emotional stress
  D. A and C
  E. all of the above

E is correct.
Each of these may precipitate angina.

5.071 Descriptions of angina frequently include the following:
  A. a squeezing or pressure sensation
  B. a sharp pain
  C. radiation of the pain to jaw, neck, shoulder
  D. A and C
  E. all of the above

D is correct.
Anginal pain is usually dull in character.

5.072 Patients with angina and an acute MI:
  A. almost always have characteristic ECG changes
  B. never have characteristic ECG changes
  C. sometimes have no ECG changes in the earlier stages
  D. frequently have no ECG changes ever, even after severe MI
  E. C and D

C is correct.
Unfortunately, the "myocardially infarcting" patient may not have ECG changes, and the diagnosis may have to be made on clinical grounds.

5.073 An active 28-year-old man with exertional chest pain relieved by nitrates and ECG changes may have:
  A. chronic stable angina class IV
  B. unstable angina
  C. crescendo angina
  D. variant angina

D is correct.
Also called Prinzmetal's angina.

5.074 The diagnosis of acute MI is established by:
  A. history, ECG changes, and CPK-MB
  B. history, ectopy, and CPK-MM
  C. history, ECG changes, and CPK-MM
  D. PE, ECG changes, and CPK-MB

A is correct.
When you are lucky.

5.075 Complications of acute MI may include:
    A. CAD, dysrhythmias, angina, myocardial
       aneurysm, VSD, papillary muscle rupture
    B. CHF, dysrhythmias (primarily atrial), angina,
       myocardial aneurysm, VSD, papillary muscle
       rupture
    C. CHF, dysrhythmias, angina, aortic aneurysm,
       tetralogy of Fallot, papillary muscle rupture
    D. CHF, dysrhythmias (primarily ventricular),
       angina, myocardial aneurysm, VSD, papillary
       muscle rupture
    E. CHF, dysrhythmias, angina, myocardial aneurysm,
       VSD, hypertension

D is correct.
Depending on the extent and location of the myocardial damage.

5.076 The MOST common clinical manifestation of CAD is:
    A. angina
    B. acute MI
    C. CHF
    D. claudication
    E. hypertension

A is correct.
The most common symptom of CAD is angina. Many patients will have acute MI eventually or even sudden death initially as well. CHF is a common sequela of MI, valvular heart disease, or cardiomyopathy. Claudication and hypertension may result from peripheral vascular disease and may be associated with CAD.

5.077 Each of the following may be a cause of angina EXCEPT:
    A. ischemic heart disease
    B. aortic valve disease
    C. hypertrophic cardiomyopathy
    D. coronary artery spasm
    E. pericarditis

E is correct.
Pericarditis is inflammation in the pericardium, often viral in origin, and produces a friction-rub type pain that is not relieved by rest or improving myocardial oxygenation.

5.078 All of the following classes of drugs are used for long-term suppression of angina EXCEPT:
    A. β-blockers
    B. calcium channel blockers
    C. β_2-agonists
    D. nitrates

C is correct.
β_2-Agonists are used primarily in pulmonary disease for bronchodilatation and have no role in the treatment of angina. In fact, some β_1 effects can be produced by these agents, which would exacerbate angina.

5.079 Which of the following is LEAST consistent with a diagnosis of angina?
    A. normal ECG
    B. normal PE
    C. old MI on ECG
    D. elevation of CPK-MB
    E. ventricular dysrhythmias

D is correct.
Elevation of the CPK-MB band is consistent with the diagnosis of acute MI. Each of the other findings can be seen in a patient with angina.

5.080 Oxygen is given in an acute MI to:
    A. limit the size of the infarction
    B. relieve pain
    C. control rate
    D. A and B
    E. all of the above

D. is correct.
Oxygen will help relieve myocardial ischemia, relieving pain and limiting the size of an acute MI. It only indirectly acts on heart rate due to decreased anxiety with pain reduction.

5.081 Mr. Jones presents to your clinic, complaining of chest pains. He is a 55-year-old white male and has smoked two packs per day for the last 40 years. His cholesterol has been running 290–350 for the past 5 years despite his "low fat" diet. He had a MI 5 years ago, after which he developed episodic anginal pain for which he uses sublingual nitroglycerin PRN. He typically has pain after walking for 30 minutes or more. The pain is relieved by rest and one nitro. Lately, he notices episodes of similar pain with minimal activity or even at rest. This pain may require two or, in one case (yesterday), three SL nitro to be relieved. He is pain free and in no acute distress, but is concerned about yesterday's episode. The BEST working diagnosis listed is:
    A. chronic stable angina
    B. angina exacerbation
    C. unstable angina—rule out MI
    D. rule out MI
    E. CAD—rule out CHF

C is correct.
Mr. Jones' history suggests angina at rest or with minimal activity, meeting the criteria for unstable angina. He therefore should be evaluated to R/O acute MI.

5.082 Morphine sulfate is given in acute MI to:
    A. limit the size of the infarction
    B. relieve pain
    C. control rate/rhythm
    D. A and B
    E. all of the above

B is correct.   *vasodilate?*
MS also helps by both preload and afterload reduction, which decreases the work of the heart.

5.083 Which of the following is NOT a risk factor for deep venous thrombosis?
    A. trauma
    B. varicose vein
    C. respiratory distress
    D. inactivity
    E. pregnancy

C is correct.
Although it may result from DVT via PE.

5.084 The hall mark of vascular insufficiency is:
    A. hypertension
    B. paresthesias
    C. pallor
    D. claudication

D is correct.
"Angina" of the calf muscles, just like angina due to myocardial ischemia.

5.085 Erectile impotence in a patient with claudication:
    A. may be directly related to vascular disease
    B. is not related to the disease unless also diabetic
    C. is not related and suggests LS spine as etiology of the leg pain
    D. is not related

A is correct.
Vascular insufficiency is an important cause of impotence.

5.086 Development of leg pain at rest in a patient with intermittent claudication suggests:
    A. progression of vascular disease
    B. new collateral circulation
    C. misdiagnosis of presenting complaint
    D. new pathological process

A is correct.
To continue the analogy, this is "unstable angina" of the calf muscles.

5.087 Which of the following causes of peripheral edema is associated with pigmentation changes?
  A. lymphedema
  B. chronic venous insufficiency
  C. orthostatic edema
  D. lipedema
  E. varicose veins

B is correct.
Pigmentation of the skin is common with chronic venous insufficiency.

5.088 On exam, you raise both legs to about 60°. In a patient with arterial insufficiency, the feet will:
  A. appear dusky red
  B. flush bright pink
  C. become markedly pale
  D. maintain normal color
  E. will look bluish

C is correct.
Mild pallor is normal.

5.089 Which is NOT associated with chronic arterial insufficiency?
  A. ulcers about the ankle
  B. decreased pulses
  C. claudication
  D. rubor with dependency
  E. hair loss over the foot and toes

A is correct.
Ulcers are more typical of venous insufficiency.

5.090 Which is NOT associated with chronic venous insufficiency?
  A. normal pulses
  B. cyanosis on dependency
  C. gangrene
  D. stasis dermatitis
  E. edema

C is correct.
This may develop in advanced arterial insufficiency.

5.091 Which results in edema by decreasing colloid osmotic pressure?
  A. lymphedema
  B. lipedema
  C. orthostatic edema
  D. right-sided CHF
  E. hypoalbuminemia

E is correct.
Lack of plasma protein (albumin) decreases the colloid osmotic pressure.

TEST PLAN FOR SECTION 5: CIRCULATORY SYSTEM

Tasks/areas assessed	Hx and PE	Dx studies	Diagnosis	Prognosis	Health maintenance	Management Clinical intervention	Clinical therapeutics	Applying scientific concepts
Total questions = 91	17	23	10	3	5	6	4	23
					question numbers			
Diseases/disorders								
Essential hypertension	54,55	30–36,51	56		57		52	53
Malignant hypertension								
Secondary hypertension								
Angina pectoris	70	71	72,80	67	58,59,63,65	64,66	68	60–62,69
Myocardial infarction		23–29,73	22,78	74		79	77,81	75,76
Other ischemic heart diseases		17						
Cardiomyopathy	37							
Congestive heart failure	3,5,6							
Pericarditis								
Arrhythmias/ conduction disorders	50	14–16,18,19	20,21,45,46			43,44,47		8–13,48,49
Arterial embolism								
Aortic aneurysm								
Peripheral vascular disease	83,87,89		88	85				84,90,91
Phlebitis/ thrombophlebitis								
Endocarditis								
Rheumatic fever/ myocardial tissue and valve related	1,2,4,7,38							39–42
Venous embolism/ thrombosis								82
Varicose veins	86							

SECTION 6: DIGESTIVE SYSTEM

6.001 Tenesmus describes:
  A. fecal incontinence
  B. bright red blood per rectum with each bowel movement
  C. fecal impaction
  D. painful straining with a bowel movement
  E. rectal pain not related to a bowel movement

D is correct.
It can also refer to similar symptoms with urination.

6.002 Which of the following will make an abdominal examination MORE difficult?
  A. patient's hands behind head
  B. patient's arms crossed on chest
  C. slight elevation of patient's head
  D. pillow under patient's knees

A is correct.
This will result in tightening of the abdominal musculature. The other choices will facilitate the exam.

6.003 Costovertebral angle tenderness on fist percussion suggests:
  A. hepatitis
  B. mononucleosis
  C. pyelonephritis
  D. abdominal aortic aneurysm
  E. degenerative disc disease

C is correct.
CVA fist percussion is done to "jostle" the kidneys and elicits tenderness in the patient with inflammation of the underlying organ.

6.004 Fist percussion of the costovertebral angle is:
  A. posterior at 10–11 intercostal space at posterior axillary line
  B. posterior at 10–11 intercostal space adjacent to back bones
  C. posterior at 8–10 intercostal space adjacent to back bones
  D. laterally at 10–11 intercostal space at mid-axillary line

B is correct.
Accurate location increases the reliability of this assessment.

6.005 Palpation of the liver below the right costal margin is:
  A. always possible
  B. sometimes possible in normal patients
  C. only possible in children
  D. always pathological in adults

B is correct.
Normal variation in the size, shape, and position of the liver with breathing may allow it to be palpated below the costal margin in well patients.

6.006 In palpating bimanually for the right kidney in the right upper quadrant in a thin 18-year-old woman, you find you can trap the inferior pole of the kidney only. This suggests:
  A. normal exam
  B. abnormally high position of the kidney
  C. abnormally low position of the kidney
  D. gross enlargement

A is correct.
It is common to appreciate only the lower pole of the right kidney on palpation.

6.007 In palpating for the liver, spleen, and kidneys in an obese 30-year-old man, you are unable to appreciate any of the organs. This is MOST likely:
   A. tumor-filled abdomen
   B. ascites
   C. normal exam
   D. gas-filled abdomen

C is correct.
Abdominal exam becomes increasingly difficult as patient's become more obese.

6.008 Bright red blood per rectum usually originates:
   A. proximal to the ileocecal valve
   B. right colon with slow transit
   C. left colon
   D. anorectal region
   E. C and D

E is correct.
BRBPR suggests low GI tract bleeding, unless transit is rapid. Slow upper GI bleeding would produce melanotic stool.

6.009 A positive fluid-wave test is:
   A. normal
   B. abnormal, suggesting pregnancy
   C. abnormal, suggesting hepatosplenomegaly
   D. abnormal, suggesting ascites
   E. normal in obese patients

D is correct.
Fluid-wave test is positive when ballottement of one side of the abdomen produces a palpable wave on the opposite side, despite the presence of a midline barrier (hand); this represents significant ascites.

6.010 Associated with cholecystitis is:
   A. psoas sign
   B. Rovsing's sign
   C. fluid-wave test
   D. Murphy's sign

D is correct.
A sharp increase in pain on inspiration with pressure in the RUQ causes the patient to limit the inspiratory effort.

6.011 Associated with cholecystitis is:
   A. fecundity
   B. male sex
   C. dark skin
   D. cachexia

A is correct.
Multiparous women are at higher risk for gallbladder disease.

6.012 The psoas sign can be elicited by:
   A. a resisted straight leg raise on the left
   B. a resisted straight leg raise on the right
   C. right knee and hip flexed at 90°, then rotation at the hip
   D. left knee and hip flexed at 90°, then rotation at the hip

B is correct.

6.013 The obturator sign can be elicited by:
   A. a resisted straight leg raise on the right
   B. a resisted straight leg raise on the left
   C. right knee and hip flexed at 90°, then internal rotation at the hip
   D. left knee and hip flexed at 90°, then internal rotation at the hip

C is correct.
Pain with this maneuver is suggestive of appendicitis.

6.014 Rovsing's sign is:
   A. right upper quadrant pain with right upper quadrant rebound
   B. left lower quadrant pain with rebound of left lower quadrant
   C. right lower quadrant pain with rebound of right lower quadrant
   D. right lower quadrant pain with rebound of left lower quadrant

D is correct.
Also called "referred rebound."

6.015 Stool for occult blood becomes routine part of annual exam for:
   A. males at 50, females at 50
   B. males at 45, females at 50
   C. males at 50, females at 40
   D. males at 60, females at 50
   E. males at 50, females at 60

A is correct.
Colon cancer is one of the most common treatable cancers. It is uncommon before 50, but risk increases with age subsequently in both men and women.

6.016 Goals of the rectal exam in abdominal pain may include:
   A. ruling out bleeding
   B. assessing for retrocecal appendix
   C. assessing for masses
   D. all of the above

D is correct.
Rectal exam is mandatory in patients with abdominal pain.

6.017 When palpating the abdomen, watch:
   A. your hands
   B. the area away from your hands
   C. the patient's face
   D. the patient's legs

C is correct.
Watching the patient's facial expression helps identify areas of tenderness.

6.018 Which of the following is ABNORMAL on inspection?
   A. silver striae
   B. fine venous network
   C. pink, purple striae
   D. scaphoid abdomen

C is correct.
Pink, purple striae can be associated with Cushing's syndrome.

6.019 Which of the following is MOST likely to be a NORMAL finding?
   A. pulsations in left lower quadrant
   B. pulsations in right lower quadrant
   C. pulsations in epigastrium
   D. pulsations in suprapubic area

C is correct.
Aortic pulsations are normally felt in the epigastrium to about the level of the umbilicus.

6.020 The correct sequence of the abdominal exam is:
   A. inspection, auscultation, percussion, palpation
   B. inspection, palpation, auscultation, percussion
   C. inspection, auscultation, palpation, percussion
   D. auscultation, inspection, palpation, percussion

C is correct.
To prevent the stimulation of false bowel sounds, auscultation is done prior to percussion and palpation.

6.021 Borborygmi is BEST defined as:
   A. absence of bowel sounds
   B. occasional tingling bowel sounds
   C. "stomach growling"
   D. rare low-pitched sounds associated with hypoperistalsis

C is correct.
Can you hear the hyperdynamic bowel sounds when you say the word?

6.022 Friction rubs over the liver may represent:
   A. perihepatitis
   B. carcinoma
   C. recent biopsy
   D. all of the above

D is correct.
Although rare, they represent inflammation of the peritoneal surface of the organ due to any cause.

6.023 Normal liver dullness in the right mid-clavicular line is:
   A. 6–12 cm; male greater than female; large persons less than small persons
   B. 4–8 cm; male greater than female; small persons less than large persons
   C. 6–12 cm; female greater than male; small persons less than large persons
   D. 4–8 cm; female greater than male; small persons less than large persons
   E. 6–12 cm; male greater than female; small persons less than large persons

E is correct.
A gross estimate, but still the best we can do clinically without "machines."

6.024 A tympanic area in the area of the left lower rib cage suggests:
   A. enlarged liver
   B. enlarged spleen
   C. enlarged, gas-filled pancreas
   D. normal exam

D is correct.
Appropriate location for the gastric "bubble."

6.025 An enlarged spleen would cause a change from ____ to ____ in last intercostal space at the L anterior axillary line with ____.
   A. tympany, dullness, inspiration
   B. dullness, tympany, inspiration
   C. tympany, dullness, expiration
   D. no percussion changes related to respiration at this location

A is correct.
An alternative to palpation for an enlarged spleen that may be more sensitive.

6.026 An obese, fair-skinned, 47-year-old woman with five children has five risk factors for:
   A. coronary artery disease
   B. pancreatitis
   C. hepatitis
   D. gallbladder disease

D is correct.
Obese, fair-skinned, fertile women in their 40s are at highest risk for gallbladder disease.

6.027 Sigmoidoscopy is routinely recommended at:
   A. 60, then every 3–5 years
   B. 50, then every 5–7 years
   C. 70, then every 3–5 years
   D. 65, then every 3–5 years
   E. 50, then every 3–5 years

E is correct.
Routine flexible sigmoidoscopy has become the method of choice for early identification of colonic lesions.

6.028 Clinical features of acute pancreatitis include:
   A. intermittent, mild, epigastric pain; may radiate to back
   B. intermittent, severe, LUQ pain; may radiate to back
   C. constant, severe, epigastric pain; may radiate to back
   D. constant, mild, LUQ pain

C is correct.
Acute pancreatitis presents with constant severe pain in the epigastric area that may radiate to the back.

6.029 Lab findings of acute pancreatitis include:
   A. leukocytosis, elevated serum amylase, elevated serum lipase
   B. leukopenia, elevated serum amylase, elevated serum lipase
   C. leukocytosis, low serum amylase, low serum lipase
   D. leukopenia, elevated serum amylase, low serum lipase

A is correct.
Inflammation of the pancreas results in elevation of WBCs, amylase, and lipase.

6.030 The two MOST common causes of acute pancreatitis are:
   A. alcohol and drugs
   B. drugs and gallstones
   C. gallstones and diabetes
   D. alcohol and gallstones
   E. diabetes and alcohol

D is correct.
Drugs have also been implicated in acute pancreatitis, but diabetes has not.

6.031 The diagnosis of acute pancreatitis is NOT supported by:
   A. fever
   B. tachycardia
   C. hypotension   , ARDS
   D. respiratory failure
   E. all of the above are consistent with the diagnosis

E is correct.
Pulmonary complications of pancreatitis include atelectasis, pneumonitis, pleural effusion, mediastinal abscess, and ARDS.

6.032 The serum lipase is:
   A. more specific but less sensitive than the serum amylase
   B. more sensitive but less specific than the amylase
   C. a poor confirmatory test if amylase is elevated
   D. neither sensitive nor specific for pancreatitis

A is correct.
Combining amylase and lipase testing will show one abnormality in 80–85% of patients with acute pancreatitis.

6.033 Chronic pancreatitis usually presents initially with:
   A. recurrent abdominal pain
   B. steatorrhea
   C. diarrhea
   D. weight loss
   E. malabsorption

A is correct.
Malabsorption (characterized by steatorrhea, diarrhea, and weight loss) is a late finding in chronic pancreatitis and occurs only after about 90% of the exocrine pancreas is destroyed.

6.034 Treatments in acute pancreatitis may include all of the following EXCEPT:
   A. pain control
   B. NPO
   C. NG suction
   D. fluid and electrolyte maintenance
   E. anticholinergic drugs

E is correct.
Anticholinergics are contraindicated in acute pancreatitis.

6.035 The MOST common underlying cause of irritable bowel syndrome is:
   A. diabetes
   B. hypertension
   C. emotional stress
   D. peptic ulcer disease
   E. parasitic infection

C is correct.
Most IBS patients will have symptoms as a result of emotional stress alone, without other types of pathology.

6.036 Clinical symptoms of IBS include:
    A. chronic waxing and waning of symptoms
    B. intermittent diarrhea and constipation
    C. exacerbation in times of stress
    D. all of the above

D is correct.
All of these are characteristic, although there is a wide range of expression of symptoms.

6.037 A 59-year-old woman presents with crampy abdominal pain of relatively new onset. She is also undergoing a divorce and has had a 15-lb weight loss. Symptoms are gradually getting worse. The stools are small and narrowed, and they test positive for blood. The most appropriate workup for her GI symptoms would include:
    A. nothing since this is clearly IBS
    B. a psychological consultation to help her with the stress of her divorce
    C. a complete radiologic evaluation and colonoscopy to exclude cancer
    D. a flexible sigmoidoscopy only, then reassurance
    E. three-position abdominal x-ray to rule out obstruction.

C is correct.
The age of the patient and symptomatology mandate a careful evaluation for cancer.

6.038 Principles of management of IBS include:
    A. patient education and support
    B. diet manipulation
    C. medication
    D. stress management
    E. all of the above

E is correct.
A supportive provider–patient relationship with attention to stress, diet, and medications as needed can be successful with this difficult problem.

6.039 Specialty referral of patients with IBS is indicated:
    A. when there is diagnostic uncertainty
    B. when the symptoms are disabling and refractory to treatment
    C. when the patient exhibits serious psychopathology
    D. all of the above

D is correct.
Any of these suggests that more than primary care is needed.

6.040 Which of the following is TRUE regarding cholelithiasis?
    A. some people remain asymptomatic
    B. all patients require hospital admission
    C. all stones will be detected by abdominal ultrasound
    D. it is impossible to have gallbladder disease without stones

A is correct.
Many people have incidentally discovered stones without symptoms.

6.041 Which is FALSE regarding biliary colic?
    A. sudden onset
    B. at its worst within 1 hour
    C. characterized by steady pain
    D. localized to the RUQ or epigastrium
    E. none of the above

E is correct.
Despite the term "colic," the pain is described as steady.

6.042 Treatment of pancreatitis includes all of the following EXCEPT:
   A. fluid restriction
   B. reduction of inflammation
   C. control hyperglycemia with insulin
   D. pain relief with meperidine (Demerol®)

A is correct.
Large volumes of fluids are usually required.

6.043 Medical therapy for gallstones:
   A. is unstudied
   B. has risks that are greater than benefits
   C. should be used on asymptomatic patients rather than surgery
   D. is an alternative for symptomatic patients who are too sick or unwilling to undergo elective cholecystectomy
   E. none of the above

D is correct.
Bile acid dissolution therapy has been successful in selected patients.

6.044 Pancreatic carcinoma is associated with all of the following EXCEPT:
   A. life expectancy <1 year
   B. distant metastases
   C. high fat diet
   D. obstructive jaundice

B is correct.
Most pancreatic carcinomas spread by direct extension.

6.045 Agents that have been definitively implicated in peptic ulcer disease include:
   A. unbuffered aspirin
   B. cigarettes
   C. coffee
   D. A and B
   E. all of the above

D is correct.

6.046 A small opening superficial to the coccyx surrounded by an erythematous halo and draining pus is MOST likely:
   A. pilonidal cyst and sinus
   B. anorectal fistula
   C. anal fissure
   D. sentinel tag
   E. anal abscess

A is correct.
Typically located in this area and prone to abscess formation.

6.047 The pain of duodenal ulcers frequently:
   A. is relieved by food
   B. starts immediately after eating
   C. starts immediately after eating fatty foods
   D. is colicky in character
   E. is relieved by fasting

A is correct.
Presence of food relieves ulcer pain; empty stomachs exacerbate the pain.

6.048 The pain of perforated peptic ulcer is:
   A. gradual in onset, peaking in 24 hours
   B. gradual in onset, peaking 8 hours
   C. gradual in onset, peaking in 2 hours
   D. sudden onset

D is correct.
Patients may even be able to pinpoint the moment of perforation.

6.049 The BEST initial diagnostic study in suspected perforated peptic ulcer is:
   A. abdominal ultrasound
   B. upright abdominal x-ray
   C. CBC
   D. SMAC

B is correct.
Upright view of the abdomen shows free air under the diaphragm in 70–80% of patients.

6.050 Antibiotic therapy for ulcers may be effective in patients with ____ infection.
   A. *Giardia lamblia*
   B. *Helicobacter pylori*
   C. *Escherichia coli*
   D. *Yersinia enterocolitica*
   E. *Vibrio cholerae*

B is correct.
All of the others cause diarrheal disease.

6.051 A common complication after some types of fundoplication for hiatal hernia can be:
   A. reflux
   B. ulcers
   C. obstruction
   D. loss of appetite
   E. diarrhea

C is correct.
History of any prior abdominal surgery is an important clue in a patient with suspected obstruction.

6.052 Which is MORE suggestive of inflammatory bowel disease than acute gastroenteritis?
   A. abdominal pain
   B. watery diarrhea
   C. fever
   D. bloody diarrhea
   E. vomiting

D is correct.
Although some enteric infections are invasive and may cause bloody diarrhea, most do not, and inflammatory disease should be ruled out in a patient with bloody diarrhea.

6.053 In a patient with GI losses, a physical finding of volume depletion is:
   A. orthostatic BP changes
   B. edema
   C. bradycardia
   D. JVD
   E. increased pulse pressure

A is correct.
Orthostatic hypotension is a sensitive indicator of volume status.

6.054 A major medical therapy in ulcerative colitis is:
   A. cimetidine (Tagamet®)
   B. sulfasalazine (Azulfidine®)
   C. sulfathiazole (Sultrin®)
   D. sulfamethoxazole (Gantanol®)

B is correct.
Cimetidine is used in ulcer disease. Sulfathiazole is a vaginal antimicrobial, and sulfamethoxazole is an antibiotic.

6.055 The MOST common cause of obstruction of the appendix is:
   A. fecalith
   B. lymphatic hypertrophy
   C. lymphoma
   D. adenocarcinoma

A is correct.
Occasionally seen on x-ray, and makes your diagnosis.

6.056 A 55-year-old man presents with vague LLQ pain after eating. It is increasing in severity, and he has had one loose bowel movement and urinated once since the pain began. The MOST likely diagnosis is:
    A. appendicitis
    B. cholecystitis
    C. diverticulitis
    D. hepatitis
    E. small bowel obstruction

C is correct.
The age of the patient and location of the pain are the best clues to the diagnosis.

6.057 Hepatitis A:
    A. is almost always self-limited
    B. may be subclinical and never detected
    C. associated with prior hepatitis B infection.
    D. A and B only
    E. all of the above

D is correct.

6.058 Involuntary spasm of muscles overlying an inflamed organ is termed:
    A. rebound
    B. guarding
    C. rigidity
    D. Rovsing's sign

B is correct.
This may be difficult to distinguish from voluntary guarding by the patient.

6.059 A sentinel bowel movement in a patient with appendicitis results from:
    A. inflammation of the peritoneum
    B. increased bowel activity secondary to obstruction
    C. hypersecretion of the appendiceal mucosa
    D. ischemia of the appendiceal wall

B is correct.
The bowel increases its activity in response to obstruction.

6.060 Typical nonperforated appendicitis produces:
    A. hypothermia
    B. normal temperature
    C. low-grade fever
    D. high fever

C is correct.
Slight fever is common.

6.061 The development of somatic pain in acute appendicitis:
    A. may be RLQ if appendix is typically located
    B. may be felt in the back if retrocecal appendix
    C. may be in LLQ if appendix is transverse
    D. may not occur if appendix is protected from parietal peritoneum

D is correct.
A to C represent visceral pain in appendicitis.

6.062 Which of the following will result in altered presentation of acute appendicitis?
    A. steroids
    B. immune deficiency
    C. very young patient
    D. NSAIDs
    E. all of the above

E is correct.
Each of these may result in atypical presentation.

6.063 Perhaps the MOST important treatment for alcoholic liver disease is:
   A. corticosteroids
   B. high-protein diet
   C. cessation of alcohol consumption
   D. bed rest

C is correct.
Continued consumption will accelerate disease progression.

6.064 In the patient with advanced liver disease, hepatic encephalopathy is diagnosed by:
   A. serum protein levels
   B. stool pH
   C. serum ammonia levels
   D. clinical findings

D is correct.
Clinical neurological findings make the diagnosis.

6.065 Specific medications helpful in hepatic encephalopathy include:
   A. lactulose
   B. phenobarbitol
   C. Librium®
   D. Valium®

A is correct.
Aimed at lowering blood ammonia by trapping in the GI tract. Anxiolytics and sedatives may precipitate hepatic encephalopathy.

TEST PLAN FOR SECTION 6: DIGESTIVE SYSTEM

Tasks/areas assessed	Hx and PE	Dx studies	Diagnosis	Prognosis	Health maintenance	Clinical intervention	Clinical therapeutics	Applying scientific concepts
						Management		
Total questions = 65	29	4	3	4	3	3	5	14
					question numbers			
Diseases/disorders								
Esophagitis								
Esophageal neoplasms								
Other diseases of esophagus								
Disorder of stomach	24							
Duodenal ulcer	47							
Gastric ulcer								
Gastritis/duodenitis								
Gastric neoplasms								
Peptic ulcer	48	49			45		50	55,58,59,61,62
Appendicitis	12–14,60		56					
Constipation	1							
Diverticula			57					
Enteric infections	53							
Inflammatory bowel disease	52						54	16
Intestinal obstruction								
Irritable bowel syndrome	36			39		38		35
Ischemic bowel disease								
Small intestinal/colonic neoplasms		37			15,27			
Peritonitis	2,20,21							
Other diseases of intestines	17							
Other noninfectious gastroenteritis								

(continued on next page)

TEST PLAN FOR SECTION 6 (continued)

Tasks/areas assessed	Hx and PE	Dx studies	Diagnosis	Prognosis	Management			Applying scientific concepts
					Health maintenance	Clinical intervention	Clinical therapeutics	
Abscess of anal/rectal regions								
Anal fissure								
Hemorrhoids								
Rectal neoplasms								8
Pilonidal cyst without abscess								46
Other diseases of rectum								
Cholecystitis	10							11
Cholelithiasis	41						43	26,40
Cirrhosis	9			64		63	65	
Hepatitis	3–7,18							
Hepatoma	22							
Other diseases of liver	23							
Diseases of pancreas	19,28	29,32	31			34	42	30,33
Pancreatic neoplasms	20			44				
Congenital anomalies of GI system								
Hernias				51				
Other neoplasms								

SECTION 7: EMOTIONAL DISORDERS

7.001 Most patients with psychiatric problems present to primary care practitioners with:
   A. sadness
   B. phobias
   C. anxiety
   D. medical complaints

D is correct.
Patients with vague complaints such as fatigue, dizziness, or "nerves" often present to primary care providers looking for medical reasons for psychiatric problems.

7.002 Important elements of the psychiatric history include:
   A. medical history
   B. sleep disturbance
   C. history of prior mental illness
   D. appetite changes
   E. all of the above

E is correct.
Medical conditions can be responsible for emotional symptoms (e.g., the anxiety that accompanies hypoxemia), so a medical history with special attention to drugs is necessary. Functional changes in sleep, appetite, and libido often accompany psychological disorders like depression.

7.003 Which of the following is important to identify in the family medical history for psychiatric problems?
   A. schizophrenia
   B. alcoholism
   C. bipolar disorder
   D. A and C
   E. all of the above

E is correct.
All of these problems tend to run in families.

7.004 The psychiatrist's BEST tool to assess psychological well-being is:
   A. physical exam
   B. DSM-IVB
   C. interview
   D. mental status exam
   E. proverb interpretation

D is correct.
The mental status exam includes assessment of observable characteristics of the functioning mind. These include level of consciousness, attention, memory, orientation, and too much more to include here.

7.005 Delusions are:
   A. seeing things that are not there
   B. false beliefs that cannot be corrected
   C. hearing things that are not there
   D. unfocused feelings of anxiety

B is correct.
False perceptions like A and C are hallucinations. Anxiety is best termed anxiety.

7.006 Buspirone may be useful in:
   A. generalized anxiety disorder
   B. panic attacks
   C. agoraphobia
   D. simple phobia
   E. obsessive-compulsive disorder

A is correct.
Indicated for generalized anxiety disorders, buspirone is not a controlled substance and is not related to the other classes with abuse potential such as the benzodiazepines.

7.007 Patients presenting with disorientation MOST likely have:
   A. schizophrenia
   B. anxiety disorder
   C. affective disorder
   D. medical problem

D is correct.
Most disoriented patients will have medical problems as the underlying etiology of their disorientation.

7.008 Level of consciousness is affected in:
    A. delirium
    B. dementia
    C. organic delusional syndrome
    D. amnesic syndrome
    E. organic personality syndrome

A is correct.
None of the others listed results in altered level of consciousness.

7.009 Major intellectual abilities are intact in:
    A. delirium
    B. dementia
    C. organic delusional syndrome
    D. A and B
    E. all of the above

C is correct.
Dementia results in significant general loss; delirium does as well, but may be less so.

7.010 A 28-year-old man presents to the ER with sudden onset of shortness of breath, faintness, trembling, and nausea. He denies any precipitating events or prior similar episodes. After ruling-out of medical problems, a mental status exam identifies depersonalization and derealization. The MOST likely diagnosis is:
    A. panic attack
    B. panic disorder
    C. schizophrenia
    D. generalization disorder
    E. affective disorder

A is correct.
The new, sudden, unprovoked onset of these autonomic symptoms is typical of panic attack.

7.011 Organic diseases that can present as panic attack include:
    A. hyperthyroidism, hypothyroidism, hyperparathyroidism, mitral valve prolapse
    B. hyperglycemia
    C. ETOH or other drug withdrawal
    D. A and C
    E. all of the above

D is correct.
Hypoglycemia may produce the "fight or flight" symptoms of panic attack.

7.012 Agoraphobia is fear of :
    A. heights
    B. water
    C. public places
    D. farm animals
    E. none of the above

C is correct.
Agora refers to the marketplace. Fear of heights is acrophobia, water hydrophobia, and farm animals vegetarianism.

7.013 Simple phobia is excessive fear of an object/place that leads to:
    A. severe anxiety
    B. depression
    C. hallucinations
    D. delusions
    E. confabulations

A is correct.
Simple phobias are not complicated by these other problems.

7.014 Persistent anxiety mimicking psychiatric disorder may also be caused by:
    A. caffeine
    B. anemia
    C. COPD
    D. A and B
    E. all of the above

E is correct.
These and numerous other medical causes of anxiety must be ruled out before a psychiatric diagnosis can be reached.

7.015 Marked behavioral changes are prominent in:
   A. organic delusional syndrome
   B. organic affective syndrome
   C. organic personality syndrome
   D. organic hallucinosis

C is correct.
Organic personality syndrome may result in impaired impulse control, apathy, suspiciousness, or other behavioral changes.

7.016 Invented or distorted words used by psychotic patients are described as:
   A. confabulations
   B. echolalia
   C. clanging
   D. flight of ideas
   E. neologisms

E is correct.
Common in schizophrenics, and may also refer to new or idiosyncratic meanings of words.

7.017 Medical problems that can present with episodic anxiety:
   A. congestive heart failure
   B. hypercalcemia
   C. hyperglycemia
   D. hypertension
   E. all of the above

A is correct.
CHF can result in hypoxemia that (regardless of cause) produces anxiety.

7.018 The result of events outside of those experienced by the average individual may be:
   A. social phobia
   B. panic disorder
   C. generalized anxiety disorder
   D. post-traumatic stress disorder
   E. adjustment disorder

D is correct.
Unusually severe stresses such as war or rape can result in PTSD.

7.019 An almost continuous flow of rapid speech with sudden changes of topic is BEST described as:
   A. confabulations
   B. echolalia
   C. clanging
   D. flight of ideas
   E. neologisms

D is correct.
Frequent in manic patients. (Tim Allen would say in women.)

7.020 Repetition of other persons' words is BEST described as:
   A. confabulations
   B. echolalia
   C. clanging
   D. flight of ideas
   E. neologisms

B is correct.
Seen in patients with organic mental disorders and schizophrenia.

7.021 Panic disorders are treated with:
   A. antidepressants
   B. benzodiazepines
   C. β-blockers
   D. A and B
   E. all of the above

E is correct.

7.022 Agoraphobia may be treated with:
    A. exposure therapy
    B. benzodiazepines
    C. MAO inhibitors
    D. A and B
    E. all of the above

A is correct.

7.023 PTSD may be treated with:
    A. antidepressants
    B. benzodiazepines
    C. MAO inhibitors
    D. β-blockers
    E. all of the above

E is correct.

7.024 Recommendations for smoking cessation or maintenance of smoking cessation should be:
    A. reserved for time of maximal impact (e.g., post-MI)
    B. reserved for time when patient initiates discussion
    C. made once but dropped if not followed
    D. made at each visit

D is correct.
Studies show that eventually the message will get through to the smoker and reinforcement is important for the "quitter."

7.025 A 60-year-old man with chronic bronchitis comes to you for advice on quitting smoking. You:
    A. encourage him, as there is proven benefit in quitting
    B. encourage him despite the lack of evidence it will benefit him
    C. discourage him, as it will make his coughing more severe
    D. discourage him, as there is no benefit once COPD has begun
    E. discourage him, as failure to quit will cause him to become depressed

A is correct.
Despite his established disease, there is demonstrable benefit, such as increased exercise tolerance, to quitting.

7.026 Which of the following is a useful strategy for relapse prevention?
    A. avoiding smoking cues
    B. positive reinforcement
    C. aversive conditioning
    D. all of the above

D is correct.
These are all useful strategies for patients who have quit smoking.

7.027 The psychological model of smoking behavior:
    A. states that smoking is rewarding to the smoker
    B. supports use of nicotine-containing substitutes
    C. states smokers are avoiding withdrawal symptoms
    D. accounts for nicotine craving within hours of cessation

A is correct.
The addiction model supports these other statements.

7.028 The MOST effective strategies for smoking cessation:
    A. are behavioral
    B. are pharmacological
    C. combine behavioral and pharmacological
    D. yield 1-year cessation rates above 90%

C is correct.
Studies show that the most effective programs address both the physical symptoms of withdrawal and the behavioral rewards associated (by the smoker) with smoking.

7.029 Which of the following has been demonstrated to be effective in minimizing withdrawal symptoms?
    A. Nicorette® nicotine gum
    B. Nikoban® lobeline
    C. minor tranquilizers
    D. A and C
    E. all of the above

A is correct.

7.030 Which of the following is NOT included in the "preparing to quit" phase of a behavioral program?
    A. increasing motivation by making list of reasons to quit
    B. setting a date
    C. wearing rubber band on wrist to snap when urge to smoke develops
    D. progressive restriction

C is correct.
This is an adverse conditioning technique used in the maintenance phase.

TEST PLAN FOR SECTION 7: EMOTIONAL DISORDERS

Tasks/areas assessed	Hx and PE	Dx studies	Diagnosis	Prognosis	Management			Applying scientific concepts
					Health maintenance	Clinical intervention	Clinical therapeutics	
Total questions = 30	4	0	6	0	1	3	5	11
Diseases/disorders			*question numbers*					
Affective disorders								19
Paranoid states			5					
Psychoses originating in childhood								
Schizophrenia	3		7					16,20
Other nonorganic psychoses			8,9					
Acute stress reduction								
Adjustment disorders								
Anxiety/panic disorders			10,11				6,21,22	12–14,17
Attention deficit disorder								
Depressive disorders								
Personality disorders								15
Physical disorders of psychogenic origin								
Somatoform disorders								
Unspecified disorders	1,2,4							
Anorexia nervosa								
Bulimia								
Obesity								
Alcoholism								
Caffeine/tobacco disorders					26	24,25,30	29	27,28
Drug dependence								
Other alcohol disorders								
Altered mental status/ confusion states								
Child/elder abuse								
Domestic violence								
Rape/crises adjustment							23	18
SIDS family								
Uncomplicated bereavement								

SECTION 8: MUSCULOSKELETAL SYSTEM

8.001 The spinal level assessed by sensation on medial ankle is:
- A. L2
- B. L3
- C. L4
- D. L5
- E. S1

C is correct.
Knowing sensory levels for a few major landmarks will allow rapid localization of the level of a spinal injury/lesion.

8.002 Positive cross straight leg raises suggest:
- A. fracture of lumbar vertebra
- B. cord compression
- C. spondylolysis
- D. LS sprain
- E. LS strain

B is correct.
Cross straight leg raises are more reliable than positive SLR on the side of a radicular complaint.

8.003 A 70-year-old woman presents, complaining of low-back pain for 3 days. This otherwise well woman states she has had gradually increasing pain in the lower thoracic–upper lumbar area without radiation or neurological complaints. She denies any trauma, is taking no medications, and has NKDA. You examine her and find poorly localized tenderness in the midline and restricted ROM, reproducing her pain with movement, especially flexion. SLRs are negative and neuro exam is intact. You would:
- A. treat symptomatically with 1-week follow-up
- B. get LS spine XRs; if negative, treat symptomatically with 1-week f/u
- C. get T spine XRs; if negative, treat symptomatically with 1-week f/u
- D. get T and LS spine XRs; if negative, treat symptomatically with 1-week f/u
- E. get CBC, ESR, LS spine XRs, while awaiting orthopedic consultant

D is correct.
This patient is at high risk for compression fractures in the area noted. These may be occult fractures and be secondary to osteoporosis or malignancy.

8.004 NSAIDs:
- A. should not be used in elderly patients
- B. may have significant GI side effects including bleeding
- C. never cause renal problems in elderly patients
- D. should be supplemented with OTC aspirin if ineffective
- E. provide anti-inflammatory but not analgesic effects

B is correct.
Use all medications with caution in elderly patients.

8.005 Possible causes of low-back pain with tenderness, muscle spasm, and decreased ROM include all of the following EXCEPT:
  A. compression fracture
  B. pathologic fracture
  C. metastatic disease
  D. dissecting abdominal aortic aneurysm
  E. mechanical low-back pain

D is correct.
Lack of typical musculoskeletal findings in an at-risk patient with back pain should make the examiner suspicious of other sources.

8.006 Compression fractures in the elderly:
  A. most commonly occur in the lumbar vertebrae
  B. are more common in men
  C. most commonly occur in the lower thoracic vertebrae
  D. are treated with Harrington distraction rods
  E. are always due to metastatic disease

C is correct.
Compression fractures with anterior wedging commonly occur in this area. The lower thoracic vertebrae carry more load than the upper or cervical and are smaller and less strong than the lumbar vertebrae.

8.007 XR findings consistent with compression fracture of vertebrae may include:
  A. anterior wedging of vertebral body
  B. decreased thoracic kyphosis
  C. collars on the "Scotty dogs"
  D. osteophyte bridging

A is correct.
Osteophyte bridging is associated with arthritic changes, and collars on Scotty dogs relate to spondylolysis.

8.008 A 26-year-old male presents, complaining of sudden onset of bilateral lumbar pain while lifting. He states he felt something "give out" in his back. He denies prior injury, radiation of the pain, numbness or tingling in his feet or toes, or loss of bowel/bladder. He is taking no medications and has NKDA. Based on the history, this MOST likely represents:
  A. acute disc herniation
  B. compression fracture
  C. spondylolisthesis
  D. simple mechanical low-back pain
  E. nephrolithiasis

D is correct.
Disc herniation or spondylolisthesis usually produces unilateral pain and some neurological symptoms. Compression fractures are rare in healthy young men, and a kidney stone would be expected to produce unilateral pain with radiation to the groin with no mechanism of injury.

8.009 On physical exam for active ROM in flexion, you would normally see:
  A. lumbar lordosis becomes flat, then slightly kyphotic
  B. lumbar spine is flat, then becomes lordotic
  C. lumbar spine is kyphotic, then becomes flat
  D. lumbar spine is lordotic, then becomes flat
  E. lumbar kyphosis becomes flat, then slightly lordotic

A is correct.
A normal lumbar lordosis flattens and reverses its curvature during range of motion.

8.010 As part of the treatment for mechanical low-back pain, you instruct a patient on how to sleep in bed. He should position himself in any of the following positions EXCEPT:
  A. supine
  B. prone
  C. left side with hips and knees flexed
  D. right side with hips and knees flexed
  E. supine with pillow under knees

B is correct.
Lying prone tends to stress the lumbar spine by exaggerating the lumbar lordosis.

8.011 XRs for a patient with acute mechanical low-back pain without neurological deficits:
A. are mandatory
B. may be deferred pending 1-week follow-up
C. should not be done unless episode fails to resolve in 1 month
D. would be diagnostic for acute HNP (herniated nucleus pulposis)

B is correct.
This is reasonable in healthy patients who are not at risk for fractures or other complications to a low-back injury.

8.012 A 9-year-old boy presents with his mother, complaining of pain and swelling of the right leg just below the patella. The pain is aggravated by playing, running, and jumping. He probably has:
A. a patellar fracture
B. Osgood-Schlatter disease
C. medial collateral ligament tear
D. anterior cruciate ligament tear
E. lateral meniscus tear

B is correct.
A tender mass at the insertion of the patellar ligament would make the diagnosis.

8.013 Metatarsal stress fractures require:
A. casting
B. total nonweightbearing
C. limiting rigorous activity
D. surgical stabilization

C is correct.
Since they are usually stable, MT stress fractures are often managed with NSAIDs and limitation of strenuous activity.

8.014 Idiopathic scoliosis is MOST commonly found in:
A. elderly females
B. male toddlers
C. adolescent males
D. adolescent females
E. perimenopausal females

D is correct.
More common in males in the early school years, but much more common in adolescent females.

8.015 Which of the following is not usually helpful in distinguishing malingering?
A. Hoover test
B. straight leg raises
C. flip sign
D. floor touch test

B is correct.
Hoover test assesses effort in a patient presenting with weakness; malingerers must reduce or eliminate effort to feign weakness and therefore can be suspected. SLRs require subjective reporting of symptoms, which can be faked. Floor touch test can be performed with a disc problem, but a malingerer may refuse to perform the test, believing that he should not be able to do so.

8.016 When performing reversed straight leg raises, your patient complains of pain in the anterior thigh. This is:
A. suggestive of low lumbar strain
B. suggestive of low lumbar disc disease and warrants referral
C. atypical high lumbar problem requiring referral
D. consistent with simple mechanical low-back pain
E. normal

C is correct.
This position puts pressure on the nerve roots in the upper lumbar area, and pain in the anterior thigh is consistent with L1 or L2 radiation.

8.017 In chronic low-back pain, which could all have normal XRs?
  A. postural, osteopenia, Paget's disease
  B. metastatic lesion, osteosarcoma, spondylolysis
  C. postural, disc disease, referred pain
  D. disc disease, osteopenia, spondylolysis
  E. spondylolisthesis, metastatic lesion, referred pain

C is correct.
Osteopenia, Paget's, osteosarcoma, metastases, and spondyloarthropathy would all be expected to have x-ray findings.

8.018 Pain radiating from the buttock down the back of the leg, numbness in lateral mid-calf and lateral foot, weakness of foot eversion, and diminished ankle jerk suggest disc lesion at:
  A. L3-4
  B. L4-5
  C. L5-S1
  D. midline (central)

C is correct.
These sensory and motor innervations arise at the L5-S1 level.

8.019 A greenstick fracture is said to occur:
  A. primarily in elderly patients
  B. when bone ends break through the skin
  C. growth plates are compressed
  D. a bone bends and breaks only partially through

D is correct.
Seen primarily in children when bones are flexible, usually closed and midshaft, greenstick fractures leave an intact segment of cortex at the side that bends.

8.020 Which of the following is MOST significant when performing SLRs?
  A. pain in posterior thigh at 85°
  B. pain increased with plantar flexion of foot
  C. pain at 5°
  D. radicular pain reproduced by 45–60° SLR

D is correct.
At 85°, many patients will experience discomfort from tight hamstrings or LS strain. When the patient's radicular symptoms can be reproduced at 45–60° and exacerbated with dorsiflexion of the foot, this is highly suggestive of HNP.

8.021 All of these are found in ankylosing spondylitis EXCEPT:
  A. involvement of sacroiliac joints
  B. absence of rheumatoid factor
  C. peripheral arthropathy
  D. HLA-B27 elevation
  E. asymmetric changes in spine

E is correct.
AS is characterized by symmetric sacroiliitis.

8.022 An elevated ESR (sed rate) in a patient with low-back pain is:
  A. a nonspecific indication of inflammation
  B. specific for tumor
  C. suggestive of osteoporosis
  D. common with mechanical low-back pain
  E. specific for metastases

A is correct.
The elevated ESR suggests an inflammatory process and should prompt a search for some nonmechanical cause.

8.023 The defining characteristic of systemic lupus erythematosus is:
  A. production of multiple autoantibodies
  B. production of antithyroid antibodies
  C. impaired production of antibodies
  D. inflammation in the musculoskeletal system
  E. defective production of connective tissue

A is correct.
Patients with SLE produce multiple types of autoantibodies, which may be deposited as immune complexes in injured tissues, adding to the inflammatory response.

ANA, Anti ds DNA,

8.024 SLE may be triggered by:
   A. drugs
   B. UV light
   C. NSAIDs
   D. A and B
   E. all of the above

E is correct.
The stimulus probably differs among patients, but all of the above have been implicated.

8.025 The epidemiology of SLE demonstrates a pattern of onset at:
   A. birth, peak 1–3 years, 10 women:1 man, more common in blacks
   B. any age, peak 13–40 years, 10 women:1 man, more common in blacks
   C. any age, peak 13–40 years, 1 woman:10 men, more common in blacks
   D. any age, peak 13–40 years, 10 women:1 man, more common in whites
   E. menopause, peak 63–70 years, 10 women:1 man, more common in blacks

B is correct.
Highest risk therefore in black women in teens to 40s.

8.026 Most (>60%) patients with SLE present with:
   A. musculoskeletal complaints, malar rash, and anemia
   B. constitutional complaints, malar rash, and anemia
   C. constitutional complaints, musculoskeletal complaints, and anemia
   D. constitutional and musculoskeletal complaints, and malar rash
   E. constitutional and musculoskeletal complaints, malar rash, and anemia

E is correct.
Most patients have these four manifestations, though numerous others are possible.

8.027 Treatments found useful in the management of SLE include:
   A. NSAIDs, steroids
   B. NSAIDs, steroids, antimalarials, cytotoxics
   C. NSAIDs, steroids, cytotoxics , anticoagulants
   D. all of the above

D is correct.
All of the above may be used, depending on the manifestations and severity of the disease in the individual patient.

8.028 Osteoarthritis is characterized by:
   A. degeneration of articular cartilage and reactive bone formation
   B. degeneration of existing bone and reactive new bone formation
   C. degeneration of articular cartilage
   D. degeneration of synovium and reactive bone formation
   E. inflammation of synovial linings, swelling, and effusions

A is correct.

8.029 Finger involvement in osteoarthritis affects:
   A. primarily DIPs, producing Bouchard's nodes, sometimes PIPs and mistaken for RA
   B. primarily PIPs, producing Heberden's nodes, sometimes DIPs and mistaken for RA
   C. DIPs, producing Heberden's nodes, never PIPs
   D. primarily DIPs, producing Heberden's nodes, sometimes PIPs and mistaken for RA

D is correct.

8.030 OA in the hip can be diagnosed as reliably as by XR by demonstrating:
   A. loss of internal rotation during flexion
   B. loss of external rotation during flexion
   C. loss of internal rotation during adduction
   D. loss of external rotation during abduction

A is correct.
This is the earliest demonstrable change in the PE in a patient with OA

8.031 Patients with DJD may benefit from:
   A. physical therapy
   B. rest, heat
   C. exercise
   D. occupational therapy
   E. all of the above

E is correct.
All of these modalities can be utilized to benefit patients with OA.

8.032 The mainstay of therapy in OA is:
   A. steroids
   B. NSAIDs
   C. narcotics
   D. antimetabolites
   E. gold salts

B is correct.
The safest, most effective agents we have for OA are the NSAIDs.

8.033 In the grading of muscle strength, active movement of the body part with gravity eliminated would be graded as:
   A. 1/5
   B. 2/5
   C. 3/5
   D. 4/5
   E. 5/5

B is correct.
Muscle strength is graded from no movement (0) to active movement against full resistance without fatigue (5).

8.034 A 28-year-old man presents after falling on an icy sidewalk, landing on extended hands. He has ecchymosis and edema of the wrist. On physical exam, you palpate snuffbox tenderness. Which of the carpal bones is most likely fractured in this patient?
   A. trapezium
   B. navicular (scaphoid)
   C. capitate
   D. trapezoid
   E. hamate

B is correct.
The most commonly fractured carpal bone.

8.035 Signs and symptoms of carpal tunnel syndrome include all of the following EXCEPT:
   A. a positive Tinel's sign
   B. a positive Phalen's sign
   C. atrophy of the thenar eminence
   D. numbness and tingling in the fourth and fifth digits

D is correct.
Symptoms of paresthesias in carpal tunnel are due to median nerve pressure, so they are noted in the palmar aspect of the 1st–3rd fingers and part of the 4th.

8.036 All of the following statements are true about lordosis of the lumbar spine EXCEPT:
- A. everyone normally has a lordotic curve in the lumbar region
- B. lordosis is increased in pregnancy
- C. lordosis is increased by weak abdominal muscles
- D. lordosis is decreased by paravertebral muscle spasms
- E. lordosis is decreased by obesity

E is correct.
Obesity and weakened abdominal muscles often go together; even so, the extra abdominal weight will increase the normal lordosis.

8.037 All of the following would be suggestive of rheumatoid arthritis EXCEPT:
- A. positive rheumatoid factor
- B. elevated C-reactive protein
- C. joint tenderness and swelling
- D. unilateral joint involvement

D is correct.
RA tends to be symmetrical.

8.038 A patient with an injury of the left sternocleidomastoid muscle will have most pain and difficulty with which of the following movements?
- A. lateral rotation of the head to the left
- B. lateral rotation of the head to the right
- C. extension of the head
- D. lateral bending of the head to the left

B is correct.
This should maximally stress the left SCM.

8.039 A patient presents to the ED after being involved in a motor vehicle accident. The patient complains of pain in the neck and chest. Vital signs are stable. An appropriate course for initial action would include:
- A. check the patient's gait
- B. check for passive range of motion of the cervical spine
- C. do Romberg's test
- D. immobilize the spine until a negative cervical spine x-ray is obtained
- E. order formal C-spine series in x-ray department

D is correct.
In a patient with neck pain and a significant mechanism of injury, the spine should be immobilized at least until a cross-table lateral C-spine film is cleared. (Usually done portable in ED.)

8.040 All of the following functions are controlled by the C5 nerve root EXCEPT:
- A. triceps reflex
- B. sensory perception of the lateral arm
- C. deltoid function
- D. biceps reflex

A is correct.
The triceps reflex is enervated at the C6-8 levels.

8.041 In a patient with narrowing of the facet joints in the cervical spine, what changes would you expect on the cervical compression–distraction test?
- A. pain will decrease on the compression component and increase on the distraction component
- B. pain will increase on the compression component and increase on the distraction component
- C. pain will increase on the compression component and decrease on the distraction component
- D. pain will decrease on the compression component and decrease on the distraction component

C is correct.
Compression should increase nerve root compression and pain; distraction should relieve the pressure/pain.

8.042 Which muscle is controlled by S1?
    A. iliopsoas
    B. tibialis anterior
    C. gastrocnemius
    D. extensor hallucis longus
    E. quadriceps

C is correct.
Ankle plantar flexion.

8.043 Crepitus is felt in the knee joint. This indicates:
    A. ligamentous laxity
    B. presence of joint effusion
    C. roughening of articular surface
    D. a sprain
    E. a strain

C is correct.
Although injured ligaments may feel crepitant as well, it is most indicative of alterations in the articulating cartilage, leading to loss of the smooth, sliding motion.

8.044 Which arm fracture is MOST at risk for associated neurovascular injury?
    A. radial styloid fracture
    B. Colles' fracture
    C. greenstick radial/ulnar fractures
    D. midshaft humeral fracture
    E. radial head fracture

D is correct.
The neurovascular bundle in the upper arm lies closely along the shaft of the humerus.

8.045 A patient with a strain has injured primarily _____ tissues.
    A. muscle
    B. tendon
    C. ligament
    D. bone
    E. articular cartilage

A is correct.

8.046 A patient has a positive drop arm test. This indicates an injury of the:
    A. deltoid
    B. rotator cuff (supraspinatus)
    C. acromioclavicular joint
    D. glenohumeral articulation

B is correct.
Patients with rotator cuff tears will have difficulty holding their shoulder in abduction and will not be able to resist downward pressure in that position.

8.047 On the knee exam, the patient complains of pain along the medial joint line that is increased with varus stress and decreased with valgus. No gaping of the joint is noted on varus or valgus stress. This indicates an injury of the:
    A. lateral collateral ligament
    B. medial collateral ligament
    C. lateral meniscus
    D. medial meniscus

D is correct.
Varus stress compresses the medial meniscus, increasing pain when it is injured. There is no instability or pain on stretching the MCLs (valgus stress) and no pain at the lateral side of the knee.

8.048 On the knee exam, you note gaping of the joint with valgus stress. This may indicate an injury of the:
    A. lateral collateral ligament
    B. medial collateral ligament
    C. lateral meniscus
    D. medial meniscus

B is correct.
This suggests instability, but some degree may be normal for a patient, so be sure to compare it with the other side and ask about old injuries (like clipping).

8.049 On Lachman's test, you note movement of the tibia anteriorly. This indicates a laxity of the:
- A. anterior cruciate ligament
- B. posterior cruciate ligament
- C. medial collateral ligament
- D. lateral collateral ligament

A is correct.
As in 8.048, compare both sides.

8.050 On Apley's compression and distraction test, the patient complains of pain with distraction. The pain is greatest on the medial side. The injury MOST likely involves the:
- A. medial meniscus
- B. lateral meniscus
- C. lateral collateral ligament
- D. medial collateral ligament
- E. patellar tendon

D is correct.
Apley's test aggravates meniscal injuries on compression and ligamentous injuries on distraction.

8.051 A patient presents, complaining of weakness in the left leg. When the patent attempts to lift his left leg in the Hoover test, there is no movement of the leg, and there are no changes in the pressure of the right heel. The patient is able to lift his right leg without difficulty. The MOST likely diagnosis is:
- A. herniation of a lumbar disc compressing nerves on the left side
- B. myopathy
- C. peripheral neuropathy
- D. spina bifida
- E. malingering

E is correct.
With the patient supine, cup your hands behind the patient's heels and have him "try to lift" the weak leg. The effort to lift the "weak" left leg is felt as downward pressure of the right heel in your hand; if there is no pressure, then the patient is not trying.

8.052 On the straight leg raise exam, the patient reports pain radiating down his right leg along the lateral aspect of his lower thigh to his patella. You suspect a herniated disc. Which nerve root is MOST probably being compressed?
- A. L2
- B. L3
- C. L4
- D. L5
- E. S1

C is correct.
This is the L4 dermatome distribution.

8.053 A person who has an increased thoracic forward bend has an increased:
- A. lordosis
- B. scoliosis
- C. kyphosis
- D. list
- E. gibbus

C is correct.
Some thoracic kyphosis is normal.

8.054 An injury to a ligament is called a:
- A. strain
- B. sprain
- C. fracture
- D. contusion
- E. abrasion

B is correct.
So when a patient tells you the old injury was "much worse than a sprain, I partially tore a ligament," you will....

8.055 Which of the following is LEAST likely to result in decreased passive ROM of the neck?
    A. meningitis
    B. muscle spasm
    C. degenerative disease of the spine
    D. swollen lymph nodes

D is correct.
While tender, they should not interfere with passive ROM.

8.056 Which of the following muscles is part of the rotator cuff?
    A. rhomboid minor
    B. subscapularis
    C. deltoid
    D. biceps

B is correct.

8.057 Signs suggestive of scoliosis include all of the following EXCEPT:
    A. one shoulder is higher than the other
    B. one scapula is more prominent than the other
    C. one hip is higher than the other
    D. lateral curvature is present in the spine
    E. anterior slippage of the affected vertebral body

E is correct.
Anterior slippage of a vertebral body is found in spondylolisthesis.

8.058 The Salter-Harris fracture class that appears normal on x-ray is:
    A. I
    B. II
    C. III
    D. IV
    E. V

A is correct.
A nondisplaced fracture through the growth plate is indistinguishable from a normal bone on x-ray. It is classified as a Salter-Harris I fracture.

8.059 Tinel's test is used to assess the____ nerves:
    A. radial and ulnar
    B. radial and median
    C. median and ulnar
    D. brachial and median

C is correct.
Use a reflex hammer to tap over the area of the nerve in the wrist or elbow to reproduce symptoms of impingement.

8.060 An 18-year-old male complains of knee pain secondary to a clipping injury in football, with pain in the medial aspect of the knee joint and no obvious swelling. The BEST way to check this patient for effusion is:
    A. McMurray's test
    B. ballottement
    C. Apley's test
    D. Lachman's test
    E. bulge sign

E is correct.
Milking the joint concentrates the fluid, and a bulge appears when pressure is applied to one side of the joint with even a minimal effusion.

8.061 An 18-year-old male complains of knee pain secondary to a clipping injury in football, with pain in the medial aspect of the knee joint an no obvious swelling. The BEST way to check this patient for stability of the anterior cruciate is:
    A. McMurray's test
    B. ballottement
    C. Apley's test
    D. Lachman's test
    E. bulge sign

D is correct.
Lachman's is the best available test for cruciate ligament stability.

8.062 Assessing the full active ROM of the shoulder involves:
  A. Apley's scratch test
  B. Tinel's sign
  C. Phalen's test
  D. McMurray's test
  E. Ortolani's click test

A is correct.
Have the patient scratch the opposite shoulder as far as possible, reaching across first in front, then behind the head, then posteriorly from below.

8.063 Assessing for congenital hip dislocation involves:
  A. Apley's scratch test
  B. Tinel's sign
  C. Phalen's test
  D. McMurray's test
  E. Ortolani's click test

E is correct.
"Winging out" the hips produces a palpable click in an infant with congenital dislocations.

8.064 In performing the straight leg raise test, dorsiflexion of the foot aggravates your patient's low-back pain. This suggests:
  A. malingering
  B. tight hamstrings
  C. herniated disc
  D. transverse process fracture
  E. spondylolysis

C is correct.
This increases the stretch on the nerves and aggravates the symptoms of a herniated disc.

8.065 You are evaluating a patient who struck his right knee on the dash while a passenger in the front seat of a car that was rear-ended. He was not wearing a seatbelt but denies other injury. The right foot is pale compared to the left; this suggests the possibility of:
  A. fracture of the patella
  B. fracture of the tibia
  C. tear of medial meniscus
  D. vascular compromise
  E. tear of the lateral collateral ligaments

D is correct.
Posterior dislocations of the tibia, as occur in knee-to-dash injuries, are prone to vascular compromise.

8.066 Placing weights in both hands with arms at the patient's side assesses stability of the:
  A. wrist
  B. sternoclavicular joint
  C. radial-ulnar joint
  D. glenohumeral joint
  E. acromioclavicular joint

E is correct.
AC joint instability can be measured by size of the gap produced when x-rays are taken in this way.

8.067 Apprehension tests are used to evaluate chronically dislocating _____ joints.
  A. hip and patellofemoral
  B. glenohumeral and patellofemoral
  C. hip and glenohumeral
  D. patellofemoral and DIP
  E. DIP and PIP

B is correct.
A patient with chronically dislocating patella or shoulder will resist movements that reproduce the mechanism of dislocation (apprehension tests).

8.068 Immediate swelling in an injured joint suggests:
  A. edema
  B. bleeding
  C. fracture
  D. chronic inflammation
  E. sprain

B is correct.
It may be associated with sprain or fracture, but in order to swell immediately, there must be bleeding in the injury. Edema takes time to develop.

8.069 Point tenderness in an injured area suggests:
    A. fracture
    B. strain
    C. sprain
    D. bleeding
    E. edema

A is correct.
Without pseudarthrosis, gross deformity, or an open fracture with visible broken bone, point tenderness over bone is the best sign of fracture on PE.

8.070 The MOST commonly injured ligament in the ankle is the:
    A. deltoid
    B. anterior talofibular
    C. medial talofibular
    D. posterior talofibular
    E. talocalcaneal

B is correct.
With inversion injuries accounting for the vast majority of ankle sprains. The anterior ligament is in a location to receive the abnormal stresses first.

8.071 A positive patellar grind test suggests:
    A. sprain
    B. strain
    C. chondromalacia patellae
    D. anterior cruciate tear
    E. recurrent dislocation of patella

C is correct.
This is elicited crepitance.

8.072 In a patient with knee pain, associated erythema may indicate any of the following EXCEPT:
    A. pyogenic infection
    B. recent heat application
    C. recent ice application
    D. bleeding
    E. cellulitis

D is correct.
Ecchymosis and/or effusion would be associated with bleeding.

8.073 A 30-year-old man with low-back pain for 2 years presents to your office, stating that his pain is unbearable and he cannot get in touch with his PMD who routinely prescribes Percodan® (a narcotic) for his pain. Your differential should include all of the following EXCEPT:
    A. musculoskeletal low-back pain
    B. degenerative disc disease
    C. aortic aneurysm
    D. spondyloarthropathy
    E. drug abuse

C is correct.
Thirty-year-olds do not have dissecting aneurysms but may have drug problems.

8.074 An 18-year-old basketball player jumped up and came down on another player's foot, forcing his right ankle to invert. He heard and felt a "pop." He has not been able to bear weight on the foot since (4 hours). He MOST likely has:
    A. first-degree sprain of the deltoid ligament
    B. first-degree sprain of the anterior talofibular ligament
    C. avulsion fracture of the tibial malleolus
    D. avulsion fracture of the fibula
    E. greenstick fracture of the head of the fibula

D is correct.
Athletes with first-degree sprains typically continue to bear weight (especially if the game isn't over). With this MOI, an avulsion fracture of the fibula is the most likely fracture.

8.075 An overhang in the thoracic spine that suggests anterior compression of a vertebra is called a:

A. list
B. traumatic scoliosis
C. kyphosis
D. gibbus
E. spondylolysis

D is correct.
Gibbet as in hangman.

TEST PLAN FOR SECTION 8: MUSCULOSKELETAL SYSTEM

Tasks/areas assessed	Hx and PE	Dx studies	Diagnosis	Prognosis	Management Health maintenance	Management Clinical intervention	Management Clinical therapeutics	Applying scientific concepts
Total questions = 75	30	10	3	0	2	3	4	23
					question numbers			
Diseases/disorders								
Acute and chronic osteomyelitis								
Developmental problems	12,63							
Joint effusion								
Ganglion/cyst of synovium/tendon/bursa	55							
Myalgia/myositis	46,60–62							
Joint pain								56,68,70,72
Limb pain								45,69
Synovitis/tenosynovitis								
Other bursitis diseases								
Other diseases of muscles/ligaments/fascia	33,38,48–50							54
Other disorders of bone and cartilage	43,47,71	17						
Back sprain	8	11	2		10			
Contusion of back	15							9
Disorders of back	5,16,20,64	22	73					1,36,51,52
Kyphoscoliosis/scoliosis	53,57							14
Spinal stenosis	41							
Spondylosis								21
Osteoarthritis and arthropathies	29	30				31	32	28

(continued on next page)

TEST PLAN FOR SECTION 8 (continued)

Tasks/areas assessed	Hx and PE	Dx studies	Diagnosis	Prognosis	Management			Applying scientific concepts
					Health maintenance	Clinical intervention	Clinical therapeutics	
Closed fractures of hand phalanges								
Dislocations/separations	67	66						65
Fracture of neck of femur								
Fracture of vertebral column	18	40,75				39		42
Various fractures of foot/leg/arm		58	74				13	19,34,44
Various contusions of head/trunk/limbs								
Rheumatoid arthritis								37
Various collagen disorders	24	26			25		27	23
Other nonarthritic rheumatisms								
Pathologic fracture (osteoporosis)		7				3	4	6
Carpal tunnel syndrome	35							
Rotator cuff syndrome	59							
Temporomandibular joint disorders								
Various sprains/strains								

SECTION 9: SKIN AND SUBCUTANEOUS TISSUE

9.001 The appendages of skin include:
   A. hair, nails, sebaceous and eccrine glands
   B. hair, nails, eccrine and sweat glands
   C. nails, eccrine and apocrine glands
   D. hair, nails, sebaceous and sweat glands
   E. hair, sebaceous, eccrine, and apocrine glands

D is correct.
The hair, nails, and sebaceous and all sweat glands are considered skin appendages. The apocrine and eccrine glands are two types of sweat glands.

9.002 Causes of brown color changes in skin may include:
   A. sunlight, pregnancy, Addison's disease
   B. hemochromatosis, Addison's disease, polycythemia
   C. pituitary tumors, hemochromatosis, vitiligo
   D. phenylketonuria, sunlight, pregnancy
   E. pituitary tumors, vitiligo, polycythemia

A is correct.
Sunlight, pregnancy, Addison's disease, and some pituitary tumors may all result in deposition of melanin and therefore brown color changes. Hemochromatosis causes both melanin and hemosiderin deposition, resulting in grayish-tan or bronze color changes. Polycythemia causes reddish-blue changes. Vitiligo is acquired loss of melanin and causes depigmentation of skin, as does phenylketonuria.

9.003 The MOST common cause of bullae on the skin is:
   A. systemic lupus erythematosus
   B. bullous pemphigoid
   C. allergic contact dermatitis
   D. impetigo

D is correct.
Impetigo, an infectious process, is much more common than immunologically mediated disorders like lupus or pemphigoid. Allergic contact dermatitis would require both a sensitivity in the patient and an exposure to an antigenically active agent, such as poison ivy. This is common in general but does not often present with bullae.

9.004 Blackheads are:
   A. comedones
   B. asteatosis
   C. pseudoscars
   D. senile purpura
   E. senile lentigines

A is correct.
Specifically, these are open comedones seen in common acne. Asteatosis is dry skin. Pseudoscars are whitish, depigmented patches. Senile purpura are vascular lesions from leaky capillaries, and lentigines are commonly referred to as liver spots. These lesions are all associated with aging.

9.005 A large (>1 cm) flat, nonpalpable primary lesion is:
   A. crust
   B. erosion
   C. scale
   D. ulcer
   E. patch

E is correct.
Crusting, erosion, scaling, and ulceration are all changes that occur in primary lesions and are therefore classified as secondary lesions.

9.006 Circumscribed superficial elevations filled with fluid include:
    A. macules, patches, erosions
    B. papules, plaques, and nodules
    C. nodules, tumors, wheals
    D. vesicles, bullae, pustules
    E. fissure, crust, scale

D is correct.
Fluid-filled lesions are classified as vesicles (small with clear fluid), pustules (pus-filled), or bullae (large with clear fluid).

9.007 The early lesion of chicken pox evolves from a papule to a(n):
    A. ulcer
    B. pustule
    C. vesicle
    D. bulla
    E. erosion

C is correct.
The chicken pox lesion begins as an erythematous papule, which then develops a small vesicle filled with clear fluid. It may or may not progress to a pustule before crusting over.

9.008 Thickening and roughening with increased visibility of normal furrows describe:
    A. keloid
    B. atrophy
    C. scabies
    D. lichenification
    E. excoriation

D is correct.
This process is described as lichenification, as it resembles the growth of lichens on rocks.

9.009 The lesion of primary syphilis is a(n):
    A. ulcer
    B. pustule
    C. vesicle
    D. bulla
    E. erosion

A is correct.
Commonly termed a chancre, a single, painless ulcer in the genital area is the typical presentation of primary syphilis.

9.010 The MOST common type of skin cancer is:
    A. malignant melanoma
    B. squamous cell carcinoma
    C. basal cell carcinoma
    D. actinic keratosis

C is correct.
This is probably the single most common type of cancer. Fortunately, the cure rate exceeds 95%, and metastases are rare.

9.011 A "freckle" or a petechia is a:
    A. macule
    B. papule
    C. plaque
    D. nodule
    E. wheal

A is correct.
"Freckles" or petechiae are small flat lesions classified as macules. Papules, plaques, nodules, and wheals are raised. The proper term for "freckle" is ephelis (pl., ephelides). (I learned this from a student H&P.)

9.012 All of the following suggest that a mole is suspicious for cancer EXCEPT:
    A. change in size
    B. variation is color
    C. irregular borders
    D. location in an area usually covered by clothing

D is correct.
While they may occur anywhere, cancerous skin lesions are more likely to appear in sun-exposed areas of the body.

9.013 A vascular lesion with no clinical significance is:
  A. cherry angioma
  B. spider angioma
  C. venous star
  D. petechia
  E. ecchymosis

A is correct.
Spider angiomata may be associated with liver disease or vitamin B deficiency. Venous stars accompany increased pressure in the superficial veins. Petechiae may suggest bleeding tendencies or emboli to the skin. Ecchymoses are associated with bleeding disorders and trauma.

9.014 _____ may occur in some normal people.
  A. Spider angioma
  B. Venous star
  C. Petechia
  D. Ecchymosis

A is correct.
While they may indicate liver disease or vitamin B deficiency, spider angiomas also occur in pregnant and normal people.

9.015 The following dermatoses are associated with severe pruritus EXCEPT:
  A. secondary syphilis
  B. contact dermatitis
  C. atopic dermatitis
  D. lichen planus

A is correct.
Though associated with constitutional symptoms and lymphadenopathy, the lesions of secondary syphilis are not severely pruritic.

9.016 "Spaghetti and meatball" appearing mass on potassium hydroxide (KOH) scraping is diagnostic of:
  A. lichen planus
  B. tinea corporis
  C. seborrheic dermatitis
  D. pityriasis rosea

B is correct.
The mass has the characteristic appearance of fungal hyphae; therefore, it is a tinea infection.

9.017 Adult atopic dermatitis MOST frequently involves:
  A. flexor surfaces and the neck
  B. groin and axillae
  C. palms and soles
  D. intertriginous areas and mucous membranes
  E. mucous membranes

A is correct.
Atopic dermatitis in adults characteristically affects the neck, wrists, antecubital and popliteal fossae, and the area behind the ear.

9.018 The primary lesion seen in acne vulgaris is a:
  A. comedone
  B. papule
  C. keratosis
  D. chancre

A is correct.
The comedone (initially closed and subsequently open) is the primary lesion of acne.

9.019 Which of the following agents used in treating acne reduces obstruction of the pilosebaceous unit?
  A. tretinoin
  B. oral contraceptives
  C. tetracycline
  D. benzoyl peroxide

A is correct.
Oral contraceptives are not used to treat acne, but in a woman taking them, changing to a less androgenic form (if possible) may help. Tetracycline and benzoyl peroxide are used for their antibacterial effects.

9.020 The initial presentation of pityriasis rosea is:
  A. chancre
  B. herpetiform
  C. herald patch
  D. target lesion

C is correct.
Chancres are the presenting lesion of primary syphilis. Herpetiform lesions are seen in zoster and other herpesvirus conditions. Target lesions suggest erythema multiforme or Lyme disease.

9.021 The MOST common cause of urticaria is:
   A. drugs
   B. food
   C. infection
   D. cold

A is correct.
While foods, cold, and infection may also cause urticaria, drugs are the most common cause.

9.022 You have decided to do a KOH scraping of a 5-cm plaque on a patient's arm. The BEST site for the scraping is:
   A. dead center in the lesion
   B. the border of the lesion
   C. on normal skin approximately 2 cm from the lesion
   D. on normal skin at 10 cm from the lesion

C is correct.
KOH scrapings are most apt to find fungal forms if taken at the spreading margin of a lesion.

9.023 Tinea versicolor is associated with:
   A. chemical exposure
   B. food allergies
   C. wet clothing
   D. prior frostbite

C is correct.
Wearing wet clothing for long periods of time (e.g., bathing suits) has been associated with tinea versicolor infection.

9.024 Itchy, transient wheals suggest:
   A. allergic urticaria
   B. Stevens-Johnson syndrome
   C. toxic epidermal necrolysis
   D. Lyme disease

A is correct.
None of the other conditions is likely to be transient in nature.

9.025 Mortality due to toxic epidermal necrolysis is MOST often due to:
   A. sepsis
   B. anaphylaxis
   C. hypoxemia
   D. hypothermia

A is correct.
Mortality in TEN ranges from 25–70%, with sepsis as the main cause of death.

9.026 Drug reactions are characterized by all of the following EXCEPT:
   A. sudden appearance
   B. symmetrical distribution
   C. extensive generalized involvement
   D. severe, significant systemic disturbance

D is correct.
While overt anaphylaxis is possible with drug allergy, most reactions are not severe, systemic disturbances. (Try telling that to a 16-year-old with a drug rash!)

9.027 Seborrhea may be treated with all of the following EXCEPT:
   A. steroids
   B. antibiotics
   C. antifungals
   D. shampoos

B is correct.
Shampoos containing sulfur, selenium, and salicylic acid are used in treating seborrheic dermatitis. Topical steroids or ketoconazole (Nizoral®) may be added if needed.

9.028 Which of the following is caused by mechanical rather than infectious agents?
   A. erysipelas
   B. ecthyma
   C. impetigo
   D. intertrigo

D is correct.
A–C may all caused by strep infections.

9.029 A 24-year-old black man has pustules in the distribution of his beard for 2 weeks. This MOST likely represents:
  A. tinea corporis
  B. tinea barbae
  C. folliculitis
  D. pityriasis rosea
  E. acne vulgaris

C is correct.
Tinea on the face would be barbae, not corporis (on the body). However, since tinea infections do not usually present as pustules, neither of these is most likely. Since blacks are more prone to folliculitis due to short curly hairs and acne is more often chronic than acute at this age, folliculitis is more likely than acne in this patient.

9.030 Squamous cell carcinoma:
  A. is characterized by a pearly papule with surface telangiectasias
  B. frequently arises from a solar keratosis
  C. is the most common skin tumor
  D. is only found in sun-exposed areas of the body

B is correct.
SCC begins as areas of rough or thickened skin and slowly evolves into hyperkeratotic plaques. Actinic (solar) keratoses are considered precursors. Basal cell carcinoma is the most common skin tumor. While less common than those found in sun-exposed areas, SCC is found in other areas and tends to be more aggressive.

9.031 A form of melanoma MORE common in blacks and Asians than in whites is:
  A. superficial spreading melanoma
  B. nodular melanoma
  C. lentigo maligna melanoma
  D. acral lentiginous melanoma

D is correct.
These cancers occur in the lesser/unpigmented areas of palms, soles, mucous membranes, and subungual areas.

9.032 Impetigo represents:
  A. bacterial infection
  B. viral infection
  C. parasitic infection
  D. allergic response

A is correct.
Impetigo is a strep infection. There is no worm in "ringworm."

9.033 The lesions of zoster:
  A. can transmit shingles
  B. are usually across the midline
  C. can transmit chicken pox
  D. commonly involve more than one dermatome
  E. are best described as bullous

C is correct.
Zoster lesions are infectious for chicken pox, but not shingles, which is the recurrence of an earlier varicella infection. Shingles are usually distributed unilaterally in a single dermatome and are vesicular in nature.

9.034 A painful patch of vesicles on one side of the forehead is MOST likely to be:
  A. HSV-I
  B. HSV-II
  C. HPV
  D. chicken pox
  E. shingles

E is correct.
The location and distribution are typical for zoster. HSV-I and -II are generally less painful and not found on the forehead (oral and genital sites are most common). HPV causes warts, which are usually painless and located in pressure areas and on the genitals. Chicken pox is usually itchy, not painful, and generalized in its distribution.

9.035 Zoster at the tip of the nose:
  A. responds to antibiotics
  B. requires no specific follow-up
  C. requires PRN follow-up
  D. requires dermatologic referral
  E. requires ophthalmologic referral

E is correct.
Zoster involving the facial nerve may include the eye, so ophthalmologic referral is necessary to assess and treat any eye involvement, which could result in vision loss.

9.036 Warts are described as:
   A. vesicular
   B. bullous
   C. pustular
   D. verrucous
   E. comedous

D is correct.
The term *verrucous* is synonymous with "warty" and refers to the papillary arrangement of the lesion.

9.037 Patients with viral URIs treated with ampicillin who develop a rash are likely to have which viral infection?
   A. Coxsackie virus
   B. cytomegalovirus
   C. Epstein-Barr virus
   D. herpes simplex I
   E. herpes simplex II

C is correct.
Mononucleosis has been associated with the development of sensitivity to ampicillin resulting in a typical drug rash—another argument against indiscriminate use of antibiotics.

9.038 Target lesions are classic for:
   A. contact dermatitis (allergic)
   B. flea bites
   C. erythema multiforme
   D. scabies
   E. pityriasis rosea

C is correct.
Allergic contact dermatitis usually results in erythema, vesicles, and oozing and flea bites in red papules, often in groups. Scabies lesions are papulovesicular and may have burrows evident. Pityriasis lesions are macular with fine scaling.

9.039 Erythema multiforme can be caused by:
   A. infections
   B. immunizations
   C. drugs
   D. malignancy
   E. all of the above

E is correct.
These can all cause erythema multiforme. Radiation therapy, connective tissue disease, and hormonal changes may also result in this condition.

9.040 Secondary syphilis can produce lesions resembling:
   A. chancroid
   B. condyloma
   C. pityriasis
   D. all of the above

D is correct.
Known as the "great imitator," syphilis may have many different presentations. (One of my best teachers, Jack Fairbank, RPA-C, once advised me that if I did not recognize a rash, I should consider that it could be syphilis.)

9.041 Patients diagnosed with gonorrhea should be:
   A. tested for HIV
   B. worked up for hepatitis B
   C. tested for syphilis
   D. tested for *Chlamydia*
   E. worked up for all STDs

E is correct.
The behaviors that resulted in acquiring one STD put a patient at risk for all STDs, and therefore screening for all the others is indicated.

9.042 An isolated, nontender cystic lesion that drains a cheesy substance BEST describes:
   A. acne
   B. cellulitis
   C. whitlow
   D. sebaceous cyst
   E. abscess

D is correct.
Comedones and abscesses would be expected to drain pus. A whitlow is a painful herpetic paronychia, and cellulitis causes pain, erythema, and induration.

9.043 Nits are:
   A. burrows from scabies
   B. moving freckles
   C. adult scabies
   D. unhatched lice
   E. fleas

9.044 Atopy includes:
   A. dermatographism, pruritus, urticaria
   B. asthma, hay fever, eczema
   C. dyshidrosis, fissuring, crusting
   D. lichenification, scaling, cataracts

9.045 Lichen planus:
   A. typically involves the nails
   B. is nonpruritic
   C. can exhibit Koebner's phenomenon
   D. does not produce intraoral lesions

D is correct.
Nit is the common term for the unhatched louse attached to a hair shaft about 1 cm above the skin. Nits resemble tiny grains of rice. "Moving freckles" is Dr. "Hawkeye" Pierce's eloquent description of pediculosis pubis.

B is correct.
The typical patient with atopy will exhibit other allergic conditions such as asthma and hay fever.

C is correct.
Lichen planus can produce oral lesions, but the nails are not typically involved. It is highly pruritic, and linear streaks of lesions may appear at the site of skin trauma (Koebner's phenomenon).

TEST PLAN FOR SECTION 9: SKIN AND SUBCUTANEOUS TISSUE

| Tasks/areas assessed | Hx and PE | Dx studies | Diagnosis | Prognosis | Management | | | Applying scientific concepts |
					Health maintenance	Clinical intervention	Clinical therapeutics	
Total questions = 45	13	2	8	5	2	2	3	10
Diseases/disorders			*question numbers*					
Varicella	7							10
Zoster	34			33		35		
Candidiasis, mouth								
Candidiasis, unspecified								
Cellulitis/abscess of finger/toe								
Cellulitis/abscess/other local infections	29		28					32
Impetigo	3							
Mycoses/ dermatophytosis		6,22			23			
Acne vulgaris	4		18				19	
Insect bite, nonvenomous								
Scabies			43					
Symptoms involving skin/ integumentary tissue	15,24		2,21	13,14			37	5,6,8,11
Other inflammatory conditions of skin	17,26		20,38	25		41	27	39,44
Keratoderma, acquired								45
Lipoma	12							
Neoplasms			30	10	31			
Sebaceous cyst	42							
Secondary syphilis	9,40							
Viral warts								36
Decubitus ulcer								
Nails/hair								1
Ulcer of lower limbs								

SECTION 10: ENDOCRINE, NUTRITION, AND METABOLISM

10.001 All of the following are signs that you may find in a patient with hyperthyroidism EXCEPT:
  A. hyperactive bowel sounds
  B. fine hair
  C. tachycardia
  D. dry skin
  E. tremors

D is correct.
Skin in hyperthyroid patients is likely to be warm, moist, and smooth. Hyperpigmentation may also occur.

10.002 Polyuria, polydipsia, and polyphagia suggest uncontrolled:
  A. hyperthyroidism
  B. hypothyroidism
  C. diabetes mellitus
  D. Addison's disease
  E. Cushing's syndrome

C is correct.
Hyperglycemia exceeding the renal threshold results in glycosuria and osmotic diuresis. This results in two of the three "polys." Polyphagia results from cells' inability to transport the glucose into themselves in the absence of insulin.

10.003 Tachycardia, hypertension, agitation, palpitations, weight loss suggest:
  A. hyperthyroidism
  B. hypothyroidism
  C. diabetes mellitus
  D. Addison's disease
  E. Cushing's syndrome

A is correct.
Many of the symptoms of hyperthyroidism can be explained by increased sympathetic tone. Weight loss is due to increased energy production and utilization.

10.004 Exophthalmos may be accompanied by:
  A. pupillary dilation
  B. lid lag
  C. bright light
  D. exophoria
  E. esophoria

B is correct.
In a patient with exophthalmos, notice the lid lag that occurs when moving slowly from upper to lower gaze.

10.005 The characteristic facies of red cheeks, hirsutism, and moon face describes:
  A. acromegaly
  B. parotitis
  C. myxedema
  D. Marfan's syndrome
  E. Cushing's syndrome

E is correct.
Acromegaly results in prominent brow and jaw with enlarged soft tissues. Parotitis may look somewhat moon-faced but lacks the erythema and hirsutism. Myxedema produces dull puffy facies and thinning of the eyebrows and hair. Marfan facies is long and thin.

10.006 When palpating the thyroid, have the patient:
  A. exhale
  B. inhale
  C. cough
  D. swallow

D is correct.
This causes the gland to move under the fingers and allows for a better appreciation of its characteristics.

10.007 The MOST reliable way for a hypothyroid patient to monitor disease at home is to follow his or her:
   A. BP
   B. pulse
   C. temperature
   D. weight
   E. symptoms of depression

D is correct.
Monitoring weight is simple, easy, and reliable. It does not vary as much as the vital signs and is (at least theoretically) more objective than following symptoms.

10.008 The MOST important predictor or risk factor for developing non-insulin-dependent diabetes mellitus is:
   A. obesity
   B. sex
   C. smoking
   D. high carbohydrate diet
   E. sedentary lifestyle

A is correct.
The other important risk factor is family history of type II diabetes.

10.009 The therapy of choice for diabetics who frequently develop diabetic ketoacidosis is:
   A. diet control
   B. tolbutamide (Orinase®)
   C. glipizide (Glucotrol®)
   D. insulin once daily
   E. insulin in divided daily doses

E is correct.
Ketosis-prone diabetics require close regulation of their glucose. Diet and oral hypoglycemics do not permit the control needed for these patients. Dividing the insulin dose results in a smoother curve of glucose levels, with smaller peaks and less deep troughs.

10.010 Which of the following therapies does NOT have a proven place in diabetic management?
   A. diet
   B. weight control
   C. exercise
   D. vitamin supplements

D is correct.
There are no documented vitamin requirements specifically for diabetic management.

10.011 The MORE sensitive test for primary hypothyroidism is:
   A. free T_4
   B. T_4 index
   C. TSH
   D. total T_4

C is correct.
In primary hypothyroidism, TSH may be elevated before alterations in T_4-related variables become apparent.

10.012 Initiation of treatment in a patient with mild hypothyroidism should be accomplished by:
   A. starting young, otherwise healthy patients on their optimal dose
   B. starting all young patients on their optimal dose
   C. initiating therapy at the same low dose in all patients
   D. initiating therapy at a higher dose in young patients with coronary disease
   E. initiate therapy at a low dose in all patients and even lower in some cases

E is correct.
Initiation of therapy should be at a low dose for all patients: 50–100 mcg/day. This should be even lower in elderly patients and in patients with coronary disease. Dosing should also be adjusted based on age, size, and severity and duration of symptoms.

10.013 Routine screening for diabetes in asymptomatic, nonpregnant adults is:
  A. by random plasma glucose
  B. by fasting plasma glucose
  C. by 2-hour glucose tolerance test
  D. by 2-hour postprandial serum glucose
  E. not indicated

E is correct.
The cost-benefit ratio in asymptomatic, nonpregnant adults does not justify routine screening. Pregnant women and symptomatic adults should be evaluated.

10.014 The diagnosis of diabetes in pregnancy may be made on the basis of:
  A. two elevated (>140 mg/dL) fasting plasma glucose levels
  B. two elevated levels in a 2-hour glucose tolerance test
  C. minimal alterations in glucose tolerance testing
  D. 2-hour postprandial glucose >165 mg/dL

C is correct.
A and B represent alternatives to reaching the diagnosis in nonpregnant patients. However, due to the fetal effects of hyperglycemia, even nondiabetic women whose 2-hour postprandial glucose is minimally elevated should be treated for gestational diabetes. The precise threshold varies, with some arguing for ever lower thresholds of treatment. Consultation with an endocrinologist is recommended.

10.015 The BEST laboratory study of diabetic control over time is:
  A. graph of daily AM fingerstick values
  B. monthly FBS
  C. 2-hour PP serum glucose every 6 months
  D. glycosylated hemoglobin level
  E. random blood sugar

D is correct.
The percentage of glycosylated hemoglobin gives an excellent insight into the degree of glycemic control maintained in the period 2–3 months prior to the testing.

10.016 The Somogyi phenomenon is:
  A. when patients underreport their glucose levels from home glucose testing
  B. when patients require increasing amounts of insulin to maintain euglycemia
  C. nocturnal hypoglycemia followed by hyperglycemia
  D. reactive hypoglycemia following a glucose load— a prediabetic condition

C is correct.
Somogyi phenomenon may account for nocturnal symptomatology such as night sweats, nightmares, and morning headaches in diabetics. The rebound hyperglycemia that follows the insulin-induced hypoglycemia at night may be mistaken as poor diabetic control.

10.017 Important causes of worsening hyperglycemia during insulin therapy include all of the following EXCEPT:
  A. increased physical activity
  B. increased caloric intake
  C. occult infection
  D. coronary ischemia
  E. severe emotional stress

A is correct.
Increased physical activity may lead to hypoglycemia.

10.018 First-choice therapy in type II diabetes is:
  A. diet, exercise, weight loss
  B. oral hypoglycemics
  C. regular insulin
  D. long-acting insulin

A is correct.
Maintenance of ideal body weight is the cornerstone of therapy in type II diabetes. Oral hypoglycemics and insulin may be needed as well, but often reaching and maintaining IBW may be all that is necessary.

10.019 The etiology of hyperthyroidism is:
   A. viral
   B. autoimmune
   C. idiopathic
   D. heterogenous
   E. iatrogenic

D is correct.
Heterogenous (having more than one cause). Another one of the "code" words we can use around patients to hide what we don't know.

10.020 The primary physiological alteration in hyperthyroidism is:
   A. production/release of excess T4 and/or T3
   B. production of excess T4
   C. production of excess T3
   D. production of excess TSH

A is correct.
Excess T4 may be released into the blood (with normal amounts produced), or excess production may occur. Excess T3 is metabolized to excess T4.

10.021 Which of the following is NOT consistent with a history hyperthyroidism?
   A. nervousness
   B. tremor
   C. increased appetite
   D. weight loss
   E. cold intolerance

E is correct.
Due to increased metabolic activity, patients with hyperthyroidism tend to be heat intolerant.

10.022 Elderly patients with apathetic hyperthyroidism do not present with classic signs and symptoms but with apathy:
   A. and signs of hypothyroidism
   B. weight loss and atrial fibrillation
   C. hyperglycemia and edema
   D. weight gain and cold intolerance
   E. thinned skin and hair loss

B is correct.
This "apathetic hyperthyroidism of the elderly" may be mistaken for depression or occult malignancy.

10.023 The characteristic physical findings of Graves' disease are:
   A. buffalo hump and hypotension
   B. pretibial myxedema and exophthalmos
   C. weight gain and delayed reflexes
   D. hypotension and bradycardia
   E. CHF and atrial fibrillation

B is correct.
Proptosis and pretibial myxedema are hallmarks of Graves' disease.

10.024 Initial symptomatic treatment in hyperthyroidism is typically accomplished with:
   A. β-blockers
   B. methimazole (Tapazole®)
   C. propylthiouracil
   D. radioactive iodine
   E. surgery

A is correct.
Beta-blockade is useful in control of adrenergic symptoms of hyperthyroidism regardless of the cause. More specific therapy should follow, and caution should be used in patients with heart failure or other relative contraindications to β-blockers.

10.025 Leading causes of primary hypothyroidism include:
- A. Graves' disease, idiopathic thyroid atrophy, previous iodohippurate sodium I 131 Rx, subtotal thyroidectomy
- B. Hashimoto's thyroiditis, diffuse toxic goiter, previous I 131 Rx, subtotal thyroidectomy
- C. Hashimoto's thyroiditis, idiopathic thyroid atrophy, Graves' disease, subtotal thyroidectomy
- D. Hashimoto's thyroiditis, idiopathic thyroid atrophy, previous I 131 Rx, subtotal thyroidectomy

D is correct.
Graves' disease and diffuse toxic goiter are synonymous and a cause of hyperthyroidism.

10.026 Characteristic historical clues to hypothyroidism include
- A. weight loss, cold intolerance, fatigue, dry skin, heavy menstrual periods
- B. weight gain, heat intolerance, fatigue, dry skin, heavy menstrual periods
- C. weight gain, cold intolerance, fatigue, dry skin, heavy menstrual periods
- D. weight gain, cold intolerance, fatigue, dry skin, light menstrual periods

C is correct.
Weight loss, oligomenorrhea, and heat intolerance are all opposite what might be expected.

10.027 A patient with a low T_4 and low TSH likely has:
- A. primary hypothyroidism
- B. secondary hypothyroidism
- C. hyperthyroidism
- D. Graves' disease

B is correct.
The low TSH suggests that the cause of the underproduction is at a location prior to the thyroid gland, which is not being stimulated to produce T_4 as it should be.

10.028 The diagnosis of primary hypothyroidism is established by:
- A. low T_4, decreased TSH
- B. low T_4, increased TSH
- C. high T_4, decreased TSH
- D. high T_4, increased TSH

B is correct.
In primary hypothyroidism, the pituitary reacts to the thyroid's failure to produce thyroid hormone (low T_4) by increasing production of thyroid-stimulating hormone (increased TSH)

10.029 Physical findings consistent with hypothyroidism include:
- A. doughy skin, puffy face, diminished hearing, hypotension, bradycardia, carpal tunnel syndrome
- B. doughy skin, puffy face, diminished hearing, hypertension, bradycardia
- C. doughy skin, puffy face, diminished hearing, hypotension, tachycardia
- D. doughy skin, puffy face, hypotension, bradycardia, carpal tunnel syndrome, exophthalmos

A is correct.
Hypertension, tachycardia, and exophthalmos are associated with hyperthyroidism.

10.030 Which of the following is TRUE regarding normal TSH values?
   A. normal TSH is not a sensitive or specific indicator of normal thyroid function
   B. normal TSH is sensitive but not specific for normal thyroid function
   C. normal TSH is not sensitive but is specific for normal thyroid function
   D. normal TSH is both sensitive and specific for normal thyroid function

D is correct.
While abnormal TSH values are very common and may require further evaluation, normal TSH is both sensitive (few false-negatives) and specific (few false-positives) for euthyroid.

TEST PLAN FOR SECTION 10: ENDOCRINE, NUTRITION, AND METABOLISM

Tasks/areas assessed	Hx and PE	Dx studies	Diagnosis	Prognosis	Management			Applying scientific concepts
					Health maintenance	Clinical intervention	Clinical therapeutics	
Total questions = 30	8	5	3	0	3	2	4	5
				question numbers				
Diseases/disorders								
Hyperthyroidism	1,3,4,21	30	22,23			24		19,20
Hypothyroidism	26,29	11,27	28		7		12	6,25
Neoplasms								
Parathyroid disease								
Complications of diabetes		15			8	10	9	
Hypoglycemia								
Specified manifestations of diabetes	2	14			13		17,18	16
Nutritional deficiencies/ avitaminosis								
Disorders of adrenal gland	6							
Electrolyte disorders								
Gout								
Hyperlipidemia								
Osteoporosis								

11.001 Compared with gonorrhea, the penile discharge of chlamydial infection is generally:
- A. profuse, clear/white, indolent
- B. scant, clear/white, indolent
- C. scant, clear/white, constant
- D. scant, yellow, indolent
- E. profuse, yellow, constant

B is correct.
The discharge of gonorrhea is profuse, purulent, and relatively continuous.

11.002 Palpable, nontender, hard, subcutaneous plaques along the dorsal penis BEST describes:
- A. syphilitic chancre
- B. genital herpes
- C. venereal wart
- D. carcinoma
- E. Peyronie's disease

E is correct.
All of the other pathologies listed result in cutaneous lesions of some sort.

11.003 An oval or round, dark-red, painless erosion with an indurated base located at the coronal sulcus in a man circumcised as an infant is MOST likely:
- A. genital herpes
- B. syphilis
- C. gonorrhea
- D. condyloma
- E. carcinoma

B is correct.
The syphilitic chancre may resemble a carcinoma. However, carcinomas are almost completely limited to men uncircumcised in childhood and may also be nodular as well.

11.004 A cluster of small vesicles that progress to painful ulcers on the glans of the penis are MOST likely:
- A. genital herpes
- B. syphilis
- C. gonorrhea
- D. condyloma
- E. carcinoma

A is correct.
The other lesions listed are usually painless, and gonorrhea does not cause penile lesions.

11.005 Small, white, painless "bumps" located along the corona of the glans, noted by a 15-year-old whose first sexual experience was 24 hours ago with a prostitute, represent:
- A. genital herpes
- B. syphilis
- C. gonorrhea
- D. condyloma
- E. pearly penile papules

E is correct.
It is not uncommon for teenagers to panic and worry about previously unnoticed bumps after a first sexual encounter, particularly if it was with a prostitute. Pearly penile papules are a common normal variation. The 24-hour incubation period is consistent with "supratentorial" problems.

11.006 Usually on the left side in the scrotum and described as a "bag of worms:"
- A. hernia
- B. hydrocele
- C. varicocele
- D. tumor
- E. cyst

C is correct.
The bag-of-worms description results from the dilated and engorged veins of the varicocele.

11.007 Firm, yellowish, nontender cutaneous masses of the scrotum represent:
- A. hernia
- B. hydrocele
- C. varicocele
- D. tumor
- E. cyst

E is correct.
Sebaceous cysts of the scrotum are common.

11.008 Painless nodule within the testes that does not transilluminate represents:
- A. hernia
- B. hydrocele
- C. varicocele
- D. tumor
- E. cyst

D is correct.
Solid testicular masses in young men particularly and in all men in general are suspicious and should be considered tumors until proven otherwise.

11.009 Impotence may be caused by:
- A. diabetes
- B. MS
- C. atherosclerosis
- D. medications
- E. all of the above

E is correct.
All of the above are possible, but psychological causes are very common as well.

11.010 The pain of renal colic compared with kidney pain is:
- A. also felt at costovertebral (CV) angle, more severe, radiates to groin, intermittent
- B. not felt at CV angle, more severe, radiates to groin, intermittent
- C. also felt at CV angle, less severe, radiates to groin, intermittent
- D. also felt at CV angle, more severe, does not radiate to groin, intermittent
- E. also felt at CV angle, more severe, radiates to the groin, constant

A is correct.
Kidney pain tends to be at the CV angle, dull, non-radiating, and constant. Renal colic produces severe intermittent pain at the CV angle radiating to the groin.

11.011 Dysuria in an adult male is MOST likely due to:
- A. pyelonephritis
- B. ureteral stone
- C. cystitis
- D. bacterial UTI
- E. urethritis

E is correct.
Pain on urination in an adult male is most likely to be gonococcal or chlamydial (nongonococcal) urethritis. Bacterial UTIs, including cystitis and pyelonephritis, are uncommon, unless some obstructive process, such as benign prostatic hypertrophy, is preexisting. Ureteral stones produce colicky pain as described in 11.010.

11.012 Pruritus and "moving freckles" suggest:
- A. syphilis
- B. gonorrhea
- C. pediculosis pubis (crabs)
- D. scabies
- E. herpes

C is correct.
Only crab lice are visible to the eye. The other infecting/infesting agents are microscopic. Concomitant infection/infestation must also be considered, however, since these can all be STDs.

11.013 Painful, crooked erections are associated with:
  A. diabetes
  B. side effects of antihypertensive medications
  C. Peyronie's disease
  D. syphilis
  E. hypospadias

C is correct.
The penile plaques of Peyronie's disease result in pain and bending of the penis on erection.

11.014 A 20-year-old woman presents complaining of frequency, dysuria, urgency, and tenesmus for 1 day. She MOST likely has:
  A. pelvic inflammatory disease
  B. cystitis
  C. cervicitis
  D. pyelonephritis
  E. bladder tumor

B is correct.
Bacterial cystitis is a common etiology of urinary symptoms in young women.

11.015 Dysuria means:
  A. uncomfortable, painful menstruation
  B. burning on urination
  C. painful sexual intercourse
  D. mood changes prior to the onset of menstruation

B is correct.
Commonly used to describe pain on urination, dysuria technically can refer to painful or difficult urination.

11.016 A patient experiencing a simple cystitis may have any of the following symptoms EXCEPT:
  A. dysuria
  B. frequency
  C. hematuria
  D. CV angle tenderness
  E. suprapubic tenderness

D is correct.
CVA tenderness in a patient with urinary symptoms suggests kidney infection, often from ascending (complicated) bladder infection.

11.017 Which finding is LEAST consistent with prostate CA?
  A. nodule
  B. tenderness
  C. irregular shape
  D. an area of firmness
  E. a stony-hard prostate

B is correct.
Prostate and other cancers tend to be nontender to palpation.

11.018 On rectal exam, the prostate was nontender, smooth, firm, and slightly elastic, but enlarged with obliteration of the median sulcus. The MOST likely diagnosis is:
  A. normal prostate
  B. prostate CA
  C. acute prostatitis
  D. chronic prostatitis
  E. benign prostatic hypertrophy

E is correct.
Prostatitis causes tenderness, and cancer usually does not cause diffuse uniform enlargement, as suggested by the loss of the median sulcus on palpation.

11.019 Which statement is FALSE regarding the rectal exam?
   A. insert your fingertip into the anal canal in the direction of the coccyx
   B. lubricate your gloved index finger when doing a digital exam
   C. tell the patient what you are going to do first
   D. inspect the anal sphincter before beginning the digital exam
   E. ask the patient to strain before you place your finger into the anal sphincter

A is correct.
Please direct your finger toward the umbilicus; your patients will be much happier.

11.020 Treatment of urethritis in males may include:
   A. ceftriaxone (Rocephin®) for *Chlamydia*
   B. azithromycin (Zithromax®) for *Chlamydia*
   C. penicillin for gonorrhea
   D. metronidazole for gonorrhea

B is correct.
Doxycycline is useful for treating chlamydiosis in males with urethritis. Ceftriaxone is used for gonorrhea, and metronidazole is most often used for *Trichomonas* infection. Penicillin was used before the emergence of penicillinase-producing *Neisseria gonorrhoeae* (PPNG). Other options are now available for these bugs.

11.021 Symptomatic nephrolithiasis may be characterized by all of the following EXCEPT:
   A. unilateral flank pain
   B. radiation to groin
   C. proteinuria without hematuria
   D. abrupt onset
   E. colicky pain

C is correct.
Hematuria is expected in the patient with kidney stones.

11.022 Roentgenographic evaluation of the patient with nephrolithiasis should include:
   A. MRI scan
   B. abdominal ultrasound
   C. KUB
   D. abdominal CT

C is correct.
KUB should be obtained, often as part of the IVP series that should also be done.

11.023 A patient with a urine dipstick 3+ for protein should have this confirmed by:
   A. 24-hour urine for protein
   B. three separate tests on alternating days
   C. two separate tests on consecutive days
   D. two separate tests 1 month apart

A is correct.
The 24-hour urine is the "gold standard" to quantify proteinuria.

11.024 Which of the following is NOT an indication for admission of a patient with renal calculi?
   A. severe pain, nausea, vomiting
   B. inability to take oral fluids or medications
   C. fever and chills
   D. failure of outpatient therapy
   E. hematuria

E is correct.
Hematuria is common, and unless the patient is severely anemic due to blood loss (unlikely), it does not indicate hospitalization.

11.025 In the dietary management of patients with renal disease, which of the following is FALSE?
  A. some renal patients need only to limit dietary sodium and fluid intake
  B. many dialysis patients must limit their daily intake of protein
  C. some patients find it difficult to eat sufficient proteins while on peritoneal dialysis
  D. hyponatremia should be treated with a sodium-restricted diet

D is correct.
Hyponatremia is aggravated by a low-sodium diet.

11.026 Prevalence of bacteriuria and overt infection is greater in women than in men EXCEPT in the following age group:
  A. neonates
  B. preschoolers
  C. adolescents
  D. adults

A is correct.
At this age, there is no sex difference in the prevalence.

11.027 Which of the following is MOST often seen with urine microscopy in a patient with simple cystitis?
  A. red blood cells
  B. white blood cells
  C. red cell casts
  D. white cell casts
  E. hyaline casts

B is correct.
Red cells may also be seen in some cases, particularly with a hemorrhagic cystitis.

11.028 On microscopic exam of the urine, which of the following is MOST suggestive of pyelonephritis?
  A. white cells
  B. white cell casts
  C. red blood cells
  D. red blood cell casts
  E. hyaline casts

B is correct.
All of the others may be found, but WBC casts are most specific to infection in the kidney.

11.029 On microscopic exam of the urine, which of the following is MOST suggestive of glomerulonephritis?
  A. white blood cells
  B. white cell casts
  C. red blood cells
  D. red cell blood casts
  E. hyaline casts

D is correct.
All of the others may be found, but RBC casts are most specific to glomerulonephritis.

11.030 A 22-year-old woman with dull, constant flank pain, fever, bacteriuria, and pyuria MOST likely has:
  A. cystitis
  B. nephrolithiasis
  C. pyelonephritis
  D. pelvic inflammatory disease
  E. cervicitis

C is correct.
The pain has the characteristics of kidney pain, and the urine findings suggest infection (ergo, kidney infection).

11.031 The MOST common urinary tract pathogen in community acquired UTI in females is:
  A. *Klebsiella*
  B. *Staphylococcus aureus*
  C. *Escherichia coli*
  D. group B streptococci

C is correct.
E. coli is the most common cause of cystitis in the population described and has been cited to cause as many as 80% of the cases.

11.032 The following fluid, metabolic, and electrolyte problem(s) is/are found in chronic renal failure:
  A. hyperkalemia
  B. hypocalcemia
  C. hyperphosphatemia
  D. metabolic acidosis
  E. all of the above

E is correct.
A former supervising physician of mine once said, "Once the beans go, you're in trouble."

11.033 Acute renal failure is characterized by:
  A. rapid rise in serum creatinine and BUN
  B. rapid fall in serum creatinine and rise in BUN
  C. rapid fall in serum creatinine and BUN
  D. rapid rise in serum creatinine and fall in BUN

A is correct.
Creatinine and urea must be continually excreted by the kidneys to maintain normal blood levels. With acute renal failure, both values will therefore rise.

11.034 Monitoring the patient with fixed orthostatic proteinuria involves:
  A. annual BP checks
  B. annual urine dips
  C. annual BP and urine dip
  D. annual BP, urine dip, and microscopic
  E. referral with annual follow-up by nephrologist

D is correct.
As long as the patient's BP and complete urinalysis remain unchanged, further follow-up is not needed. The initial diagnosis, however, may require consultation.

11.035 The following hematological abnormality is common in persons with chronic renal failure:
  A. anemia
  B. polycythemia
  C. leukocytopenia
  D. leukocytosis
  E. thrombocytosis

D is correct.
Abnormalities in platelet function may also be seen.

11.036 Screening for asymptomatic bacteriuria is recommended for all:
  A. patients
  B. male patients
  C. female patients
  D. sexually active female patients
  E. pregnant patients

E is correct.
Even asymptomatic bacteriuria needs treatment if the patient is pregnant. We are not sure what, if anything, to do about the others, so "don't ask, don't tell."

11.037 The BEST way to assess kidney size is by:
  A. palpation
  B. KUB
  C. IVP
  D. ultrasound
  E. CT

D is correct.
Cheap, noninvasive, and accurate. How can you lose?

11.038 Drugs commonly associated with renal damage include:
  A. NSAIDs, vitamins, ibuprofen
  B. NSAIDs, phenacetin, acetaminophen, vitamins
  C. NSAIDs, phenacetin, acetaminophen, ibuprofen
  D. steroids, phenacetin, acetaminophen, ibuprofen
  E. steroids, vitamins, acetaminophen, ibuprofen

C is correct.
Steroids and vitamins have not been commonly associated with renal damage.

11.039 The MOST common cause of nephrotic syndrome is:
   A. diabetes
   B. systemic lupus erythematosus
   C. amyloidosis
   D. lymphoma
   E. idiopathic

E is correct.
About 75% of cases. (Patients are impressed when their PA says they have "idiopathic disease," but not when he or she says, "I dunno.")

11.040 The first and second MOST likely causes of gross hematuria are:
   A. infection and tumor
   B. tumor and infection
   C. infection and calculi
   D. calculi and tumors
   E. infection and benign prostatic hypertrophy

A is correct.
Calculi and BPH can also cause hematuria, but not as often.

11.041 The single MOST common cause of asymptomatic microscopic hematuria is:
   A. infection
   B. tumor
   C. calculus
   D. BPH
   E. essential

E is correct.
Also sounds better than "I dunno."

11.042 Most renal calculi contain:
   A. uric acid
   B. calcium
   C. cystine
   D. cholesterol
   E. struvite

B is correct.
Which leads to different dietary advice than a cholesterol stone might.

11.043 Renal calculi:
   A. almost never recur
   B. recur in about 10% of patients
   C. recur in about 30% of patients
   D. recur in about 60% of patients
   E. recur in nearly 100% of patients

E is correct.
A PA I worked with was advised by my coworkers to get a nephrectomy and schedule his dialysis for his days off.

11.044 Which urinalysis finding is MOST specific for infection?
   A. blood
   B. low pH
   C. leukocyte esterase
   D. protein

C is correct.
While all of these may be found, only leukocyte esterase is specific for infection.

TEST PLAN FOR SECTION 11: KIDNEYS AND URINARY TRACT

Tasks/areas assessed	Hx and PE	Dx studies	Diagnosis	Prognosis	Management			Applying scientific concepts
					Health maintenance	Clinical intervention	Clinical therapeutics	
Total questions = 44	11	11	3	1	4	1	1	12
Diseases/disorders					question numbers			
Acute cystitis	14	27						15,16,31
Enuresis								11
Gonococcal urethritis	1							
Hematuria								40,41
Neoplasms	8,17							
Prostatic hypertrophy	18							19
Pyuria and other UT infections		44			26,36			
Other diseases of GU tract	2,12,13	23	3,4,6		34			5,7,9
Other urethritis							20	
Acute renal failure/insufficiency		33						38
Chronic renal failure/insufficiency		32,35			25			
Nephrolithiasis	21	22,37				24		10
Nephrotic syndrome/nephritis	39	29						
Pyelonephritis	30	28						
Ureteral calculus		42		43				
Other diseases/disorders of kidney and UT								

SECTION 12: MALE AND FEMALE REPRODUCTIVE SYSTEMS

12.001 Which of the following women is NOT at increased risk for breast cancer?
 A. a woman with a sister who has breast cancer
 B. a woman who has been overweight all of her life
 C. a woman who had menarche at age 8
 D. a woman who gave birth to her first child at the age of 16

D is correct.
Early age at first delivery reduces the risk of breast cancer. It is further reduced as parity increases.

12.002 Which of the following women is at increased risk for breast cancer?
 A. a woman with a history of fibrocystic disease
 B. a woman who abstains from alcohol
 C. a younger woman
 D. a woman with early menopause due to surgery

A is correct.
The relative risk is 2–3 times greater in women with a history of benign breast disease.

12.003 Small accessory glands in the areolar tissue of the breast:
 A. do not occur
 B. are normal and described as Montgomery's glands
 C. are suggestive of mastitis
 D. are normal and described as polythelia

B is correct.
Young women may need to be educated that these are not "lumps" in their breasts.

12.004 Breast development exhibiting elevation of the nipple only represents:
 A. Tanner 0
 B. Tanner 1
 C. Tanner 4
 D. Tanner 5

B is correct.
This preadolescent stage is identified as Tanner stage 1.

12.005 The presence of two or more nipples along the milk line on one side of the body is described as:
 A. polymastia
 B. polythelia
 C. bimastia
 D. peau d'orange

B is correct.
Polymastia is having more than two breasts. Bimastia literally means two breasts but is not a term in general use. Peau d'orange refers to the skin changes in the breast associated with impaired lymph drainage.

12.006 Leaning forward with the arms supported is a particularly helpful position when examining:
 A. adolescents
 B. small breasts
 C. pendulous breasts
 D. axillary nodes

C is correct.
This would enhance retraction signs and asymmetries.

12.007 Which lymph nodes are NOT involved with breast cancer or included in the breast exam?
 A. axillary
 B. supraclavicular
 C. deep thoracic lymph nodes
 D. lateral axillary
 E. epitrochlear

E is correct.
Epitrochlear nodes receive lymph from the lower arm and would not be affected by a breast cancer.

12.008 The majority of breast cancers are located in which area?
   A. upper inner
   B. lower inner
   C. central
   D. upper outer
   E. lower outer

D is correct.
Careful palpation of the entire breast is important, but particular care should be taken to include the entire tail in the exam, as well as the lymph nodes.

12.009 Signs suspicious for breast cancer may include all of the following EXCEPT:
   A. peau d'orange appearance of the skin of the breast
   B. history of chronically inverted nipples
   C. a hard mass
   D. lumps in the axilla

B is correct.
Chronically inverted nipples are likely to be a normal variant. New nipple inversion is suspicious for retraction due to carcinoma.

12.010 A round breast mass is suggestive of:
   A. cancer
   B. cystic disease
   C. cancer or adenofibroma
   D. cystic disease or adenofibroma

D is correct.
In distinguishing cancer of the breast from noncancerous changes, round lesions are more suggestive of cysts or fibroadenomas.

12.011 A poorly delineated breast mass is suggestive of:
   A. cancer
   B. cystic disease
   C. cancer or adenofibroma
   D. cystic disease or adenofibroma

A is correct.
In distinguishing cancer of the breast from noncancerous changes, poorly delimited lesions are more suggestive of cancer.

12.012 Retraction signs in the breast exam are MOST suggestive of:
   A. single cystic lesions
   B. multiple cystic lesions
   C. adenofibroma
   D. cancer

D is correct.
In distinguishing cancer of the breast from noncancerous changes, retraction signs are suggestive of cancer.

12.013 Which of the following has been proposed as treatment for premenstrual syndrome (PMS)?
   A. vitamin B complexes
   B. aerobic exercises
   C. progesterones
   D. dietary restrictions on salt and sweets.
   E. all of the above

E is correct.

12.014 Annual mammography routinely begins at age:
   A. 35 (baseline)
   B. 39
   C. 40 q 2-3 yrs
   D. 45
   E. 50 q 1 yr

E is correct.
Mammography becomes more sensitive as the breast tissue becomes less dense with age.

12.015 A 20-year-old woman presents, complaining of purulent vaginal discharge, dyspareunia, and lower abdominal pain. This MOST likely represents:
   A. pelvic inflammatory disease
   B. cystitis
   C. candidiasis
   D. trichomoniasis
   E. ovarian cyst

A is correct.
Cystitis would not be expected to present with vaginal discharge. Vaginitis due to *Candida* or *Trichomonas* does not usually cause abdominal pain.

12.016 A 20-year-old female presents, complaining of white vaginal discharge and pruritus. This MOST likely represents:
   A. PID
   B. cystitis
   C. candidiasis
   D. trichomoniasis
   E. ovarian cyst

C is correct.
Cystitis does not usually present with vaginal discharge. PID would be expected to cause abdominal pain, as would a symptomatic ovarian cyst. The white character of the discharge is more consistent with *Candida* than *Trichomonas* infection.

12.017 A 20-year-old female presents, complaining of profuse, yellow-green, malodorous vaginal discharge. This MOST likely represents:
   A. PID
   B. cystitis
   C. candidiasis
   D. trichomoniasis
   E. ovarian cyst

D is correct.
Cystitis does not usually present with vaginal discharge. PID would be expected to cause abdominal pain, as would a symptomatic ovarian cyst. The character of the discharge is more consistent with *Trichomonas* than *Candida* infection.

12.018 Glands that may become infected cystic structures at the posterior-lateral aspects of the vaginal opening are:
   A. Skene's glands
   B. Montgomery's glands
   C. sebaceous glands
   D. Bartholin's glands

D is correct.
Skene's glands are at the urethral meatus, Montgomery's in the aureole. Sebaceous cysts may occur anywhere in the labia.

12.019 Negative side effects of barrier methods of contraception may include all of the following EXCEPT:
   A. toxic shock syndrome
   B. urinary tract infections
   C. pregnancy
   D. dysmenorrhea

D is correct.
Failure rates of 5–15% have been noted, as well as an association with TSS and UTIs.

12.020 A patient experiencing polymenorrhea is:
   A. bleeding between periods
   B. having periods more frequently than every 28 days
   C. bleeding longer than 7 days
   D. using more than one pad/tampon daily

B is correct.
Bleeding between periods is usually termed "breakthrough bleeding" and does not represent additional menstrual cycles, as does true polymenorrhea.

12.021 The mucosa of the vagina becomes_____ after menopause.
   A. hypertrophic
   B. thickened, dark
   C. excessively moist
   D. thin and dry

D is correct.
Sometimes resulting in atrophic vaginitis.

12.022 The MOST common physical sign of pelvic inflammatory disease is:
   A. rebound tenderness of the abdomen
   B. tenderness with motion of the cervix
   C. adnexal tenderness
   D. fever
   E. dysuria

B is correct.
Cervical-motion tenderness (chandelier sign) is not specific to PID but is virtually always present.

12.023 On pelvic exam, a stellate os suggests:
A. nulliparity
B. single uncomplicated childbirth
C. multiple and or difficult childbirth
D. multiple episodes of PID

C is correct.
Stellate appearance suggests lacerations of the cervix related to difficult or multiple deliveries.

12.024 Weakness of the supporting structures of the pelvic floor leading to retroversion of the uterus with extension into the vagina BEST describes:
A. rectocele
B. cystocele
C. prolapse
D. myoma

C is correct.
This may often be associated with cystocele or rectocele.

12.025 A backward angulation of the body of the uterus in relation to the cervix (which maintains a normal position) BEST describes:
A. anteversion
B. retroversion
C. retroflexion
D. marked retroversion

C is correct.
Because the cervix remains in a normal relation to the vagina, the body of the uterus is flexed, hence retroflexion.

12.026 A bluish discoloration of the cervix suggests:
A. nulliparity
B. multiparity
C. pregnancy
D. PID
E. candidiasis

C is correct.
On palpation, it feels soft and flexible.

12.027 Intracellular gram-negative diplococci seen on Gram stain are MOST helpful in confirming:
A. candidiasis
B. gonorrhea
C. *Gardnerella* vaginitis
D. trichomoniasis
E. *Chlamydia* cervicitis

B is correct.
The intracellular gram-negative diplos are presumptive for *Neisseria gonorrhoeae*.

12.028 Hyphae and buds on KOH slide are MOST helpful in confirming:
A. candidiasis
B. gonorrhea
C. *Gardnerella* vaginitis
D. trichomoniasis
E. *Chlamydia* cervicitis

A is correct.
Hyphae and budding cells on a KOH prep represent yeast.

12.029 Tender unilateral adnexal enlargement with cervical-motion tenderness in a woman with tachycardia, hypotension, delayed capillary refill, and pale, cool, clammy skin (shock) suggests:
A. ovarian cyst
B. ovarian tumor
C. PID
D. ruptured tubal pregnancy

D is correct.
Safe PAs say that a woman of childbearing years with lower abdominal pain has an ectopic pregnancy until proven otherwise.

12.030 A woman whose menstrual history involves onset
at age 13, irregularity for 1 year, then regular 28–31- day
cycles with periods lasting 4–6 days for 38 years, then
stopping has had:
  A. delayed menses
  B. pathological menorrhea
  C. early thelarche
  D. normal menstruation

D is correct.
This describes a normal menstrual history.

12.031 The prepuce is:
  A. foreskin
  B. glans
  C. corona
  D. meatus
  E. shaft

A is correct.
And remember to replace it after inserting a
Foley.

12.032 The first reliable sign of sexual maturation in
males is:
  A. vellus hair in the groin
  B. increase in size of testicles
  C. increase in size of the penis
  D. growth of coarse, curly pubic hair
  E. testes hanging low in scrotum

B is correct.
Vellus hair is the early, finer body hair. The
other changes follow.

12.033 A congenital ventral displacement of the penile
meatus is:
  A. phimosis
  B. paraphimosis
  C. smegma
  D. hypospadias
  E. balanitis

D is correct.
Phimosis and paraphimosis refer to
excessively tight foreskin, smegma is the
cheesy material that may normally accumulate
under the prepuce, and balanitis is
inflammation of the glans.

12.034 A tight foreskin that cannot be retracted over the
glans is described as:
  A. phimosis
  B. paraphimosis
  C. hypospadias
  D. smegma
  E. balanoposthitis

A is correct.
Paraphimosis is when it cannot be returned
after retraction.

12.035 Condylomata acuminata are caused by:
  A. *N. gonorrhoeae*
  B. *Treponema pallidum*
  C. flagellated protozoan
  D. *Candida albicans*
  E. human papillomavirus

E is correct.
Genital and other warts are caused by various
types of HPV.

12.036 Smoking tobacco or marijuana:
  A. decreases fecundity of men only
  B. decreases fecundity of women only
  C. decreases fecundity of men and women
  D. does not affect fecundity
  E. facilitates sperm penetration of cervical mucus

C is correct.
Fecundity means fertility, if (like most of my
students) you don't recognize the word.

12.037 Which childhood infection is MOST commonly associated with male infertility?
  A. rubeola
  B. rubella
  C. pertussis
  D. varicella
  E. parotitis

E is correct.
Mumps can lead to orchitis and infertility in males—a tragedy, with a vaccine-preventable disease.

12.038 Animal studies after vasectomy show an association with:
  A. autoimmune disease
  B. atherosclerosis
  C. prostatic cancer
  D. all of the above

D is correct.
Perhaps related to hormone levels? Like breast cancer in women?

12.039 Infertility in females is MOST commonly due to:
  A. ovulatory dysfunction or tubal obstruction
  B. ovulatory dysfunction or anatomic disorders
  C. tubal obstruction or thyroid disease
  D. ovulatory dysfunction or thyroid disease
  E. anatomic disorders or thyroid disease

A is correct.
Episodes of PID are associated with scarring and tubal obstruction.

12.040 Diagnosis of premenstrual syndrome requires:
  A. retrospective documentation of 6 months of symptoms with an appropriate cyclic occurrence
  B. retrospective documentation of 3 months of symptoms with an appropriate cyclic occurrence
  C. retrospective documentation of 3 months of symptoms with an appropriate cyclic occurrence, followed by 3 months of prospective documentation
  D. prospective documentation of 3 months of symptoms with an appropriate cyclic occurrence
  E. prospective documentation of 6 months of symptoms with an appropriate cyclic occurrence

D is correct.
A detailed symptom diary is very helpful.

12.041 Therapy for dysmenorrhea is primarily with:
  A. antidepressants
  B. anxiolytics
  C. lifestyle modifications
  D. prostaglandin inhibitors
  E. diuretics

D is correct.
These are particularly helpful if started up to 1 week prior to menstruation.

12.042 A 12-year-old boy who has never been sexually active presents with sudden onset of right scrotal pain without any injury. He MOST likely has:
  A. varicocele
  B. epididymitis
  C. hydrocele
  D. testicular torsion

D is correct.
Varicoceles and hydroceles are rarely symptomatic, and most cases of epididymitis are due to an STD.

12.043 Epididymitis may be:
  A. secondary to benign prostatic hypertrophy
  B. from lifting heavy objects
  C. treated with NSAIDs, scrotal support, heat, and antibiotics
  D. all of the above

D is correct.
In younger men, most cases are infectious (gonococcal or chlamydial).

12.044 Prostate exam is routinely recommended at:
   A. 60, then every 3–5 years
   B. 50, then every 5–7 years
   C. 40, then every 3–5 years
   D. 50, then annually
   E. 40, then annually

E is correct.
Noninfectious prostate disorders are rare before age 40.

12.045 Which of the following is the BEST treatment for the male partner of a woman with trichomonal vaginitis?
   A. doxycycline
   B. metronidazole
   C. nystatin cream
   D. none

B is correct.
Metronidazole is indicated for partners of women with trichomoniasis.

TEST PLAN FOR SECTION 12: MALE AND FEMALE REPRODUCTIVE SYSTEMS

Tasks/areas assessed	Hx and PE	Dx studies	Diagnosis	Prognosis	Health maintenance	Management		Applying scientific concepts
						Clinical intervention	Clinical therapeutics	
Total questions = 45	14	2	10	0	4	0	3	12
Diseases/disorders					*question numbers*			
Leiomyoma								
Uterine neoplasms								
Other disorders of uterus								
Ovarian neoplasms								
Ovarian cysts								
Abnormal Pap smear								
Cervicitis/endocervicitis		27						
Dysplasia of cervix								26,35
Cervical neoplasms			23					
Candidiasis of vulva/vagina		28	16					
Vaginal/vulvar neoplasms	6–9							
Prolapse of vaginal walls	10							24
Vaginitis/vulvovaginitis	25		17				45	18
Dysmenorrhea	36,37						41	30
Premenstrual syndrome	22		40				13	
Other disorders of menstruation								20
Menopause								21
Inflammatory diseases of breast								
Breast neoplasms			11,12		1,2,14			
Other breast-related problems								3–5
Disorders of pelvic organs	19,44		29					
Infertility					38			
Pelvic inflammatory disease			15					39
Testicular mass	31,33,34							32
Torsion of testes			42,43					

SECTION 13: PREGNANCY, CHILDBIRTH, AND NEONATES

13.001 Routine lab tests that should be ordered for every pregnant patient during initial work-up include:
   A. hemoglobin and hematocrit
   B. white blood cell count with differential
   C. serologic test for syphilis
   D. Papanicolaou smear
   E. all of the above

E is correct.
Additional screenings (e.g., rubella titer and blood typing) are indicated during this visit as well.

13.002 Signs and symptoms of missed abortion include:
   A. cervical dilatation >3 cm
   B. decrease in uterine size
   C. moderate effacement of the cervix
   D. brownish vaginal discharge

D is correct.
In missed abortion, the cervix remains firm and closed.

13.003 Typical findings of ectopic pregnancy include:
   A. painless bleeding
   B. nontender abdomen
   C. ultrasound adnexal mass without IUP
   D. negative human chorionic gonadotropin
   E. all of the above

C is correct.
Abdominal pain and tenderness are typical. Amenorrhea is followed by irregular vaginal bleeding with a positive hCG. The vast majority are tubal and would represent an adnexal mass on ultrasound.

13.004 TRUE statements about placenta previa include:
   A. pain is the cardinal sign of placenta previa
   B. bleeding is uncommon
   C. vaginal delivery is preferred in these patients
   D. vaginal exam can cause complications

D is correct.
Painless bleeding is characteristic, though about 10% may have initial cramping. C-section is the preferred delivery method and has a lower fetal mortality rate. Vaginal exam can precipitate placental separation and bleeding.

13.005 The rise in basal body temperature that accompanies ovulation is thought to be due to an increase in secretion of:
   A. follicle-stimulating hormone
   B. luteinizing hormone
   C. estrogen
   D. progesterone

D is correct.
Progesterone is thermogenic, and levels increase at ovulation; therefore, it is the suspected cause.

13.006 When the placenta implants across the cervical os, the condition is called:
   A. abruptio placentae
   B. placenta previa
   C. placental insufficiency
   D. ectopic placenta

B is correct.
In a complete placenta previa, the placenta implants so low in the uterus that it entirely covers the cervical os and obstructs the descent of the presenting part.

13.007 The uterine fundus is at the level of the umbilicus at what gestational age?
   A. 10 weeks
   B. 20 weeks
   C. 30 weeks
   D. 40 weeks

B is correct.
About 20–22 weeks.

13.008 The first perception of fetal movement occurs at how many weeks in primiparae?
   A. 6
   B. 12
   C. 18
   D. 24

C is correct.
In multiparous patients, about 17 weeks.

13.009 After the birth of an infant, the umbilical cord should be examined to determine the number of vessels. What configuration is normal?
   A. one artery, one vein
   B. one artery, two veins
   C. two arteries, one vein
   D. two arteries, two veins

C is correct.
Cords with one artery and one vein are associated with a high (15%) perinatal death rate.

13.010 A mother is Rh negative. The father is tested, and he too is Rh negative. What are the chances that the fetus is Rh positive?
   A. 0%
   B. 25%
   C. 50%
   D. 75%

A is correct.
Homozygous recessive crosses can only produce homozygous recessive offspring.

13.011 Preeclampsia is a triad of which symptoms?
   A. edema, proteinuria, seizures
   B. edema, hypertension, seizures
   C. hypertension, proteinuria, seizures
   D. edema, hypertension, proteinuria

D is correct.
Evidence of seizures would make the diagnosis eclampsia.

13.012 Postpartum hemorrhage is MOST commonly caused by:
   A. cervical lacerations
   B. retained placenta
   C. uterine atony
   D. vaginal lacerations

C is correct.
Uterine atony accounts for about 50% of cases, lacerations about 20%, and retained placental tissue 5–10%. Other causes include coagulation defects and other hematological disorders.

13.013 The MOST common metabolic disorder associated with pregnancy is:
   A. diabetes
   B. phenylketonuria
   C. G6PD deficiency
   D. lactose intolerance
   E. celiac sprue

A is correct.
Gestational diabetes occurs in about 1% of women. Routine screening is recommended.

13.014 Recommended weight gain for a pregnant patient at ideal body weight is ___ kg.
   A. 0–2
   B. 5–7
   C. 10–12
   D. 15–17

C is correct.
About 3.5 for fetus, 1.0 for placenta/uterus/amniotic fluid, 3.5 for blood/interstitial fluid, 0.5 for breasts, and 1.5 adipose.

13.015 Drugs demonstrated to be safe for use during pregnancy are FDA category:
  A. A
  B. B
  C. C
  D. D
  E. X

A is correct.
Due to lack of controlled studies (for obvious reasons), few drugs fit this category.

13.016 Expected date of delivery is MOST easily estimated based on:
  A. first day of last menstrual period
  B. middle day of last menstrual period
  C. last day of last menstrual period
  D. date of estimated conception
  E. date of last ovulation

A is correct.
Subtract 3 from the month and add 7 to the day (Nagale's rule), or use a wheel. Both are based on a 28-day cycle.

13.017 Drug classifications that can be used if indicated in a pregnant patient without consulting an obstetrician are:
  A. A only
  B. A and B
  C. A, B, and C
  D. C and D
  E. X only

B is correct.
This is what the OBs tell me. Being paranoid, I consult them for any pregnant patient requiring medication.

13.018 Teratogenic agents include:
  A. anticoagulants
  B. antithyroid drugs
  C. anticonvulsants
  D. lithium
  E. all of the above

E is correct.
These drugs all have demonstrated teratogenic effects. Due to obvious difficulties, there are numerous drugs whose effects in humans are unknown.

13.019 Which is NOT a risk factor for preterm labor?
  A. age <16
  B. age >35
  C. poor nutrition
  D. prior preterm delivery
  E. hypertension

E is correct.
Though it is a risk factor for intrauterine growth retardation.

13.020 Preterm labor occurs:
  A. any time before 40 weeks
  B. any time before 36 weeks
  C. between 20 and 40 weeks
  D. between 20 and 36 weeks
  E. before 20 weeks

D is correct.
Regular painful uterine contractions leading to effacement/dilatation between weeks 20 and 36.

13.021 The primary metabolic derangements in fetal distress are:
  A. hyperglycemia and alkalosis
  B. hypercalcemia and hyperglycemia
  C. hypokalemia and hypoglycemia
  D. hypoglycemia and hypoxia
  E. hypoxia and acidosis

D is correct.
Resulting from many possible causes, permanent injury or death may ensue.

13.022 Premature separation of the placenta from the uterus it is termed:
- A. premature rupture of membranes
- B. placenta previa
- C. abruption
- D. prolapse cord
- E. eclampsia

C is correct.
Pain is experienced, but bleeding may or may not be obvious.

13.023 Vaginal birth after C-section may lead to:
- A. premature rupture of membranes
- B. placenta previa
- C. abruption
- D. prolapse cord
- E. uterine rupture

E is correct.
Dehiscence of the incision is undiagnosed silent separation of the scar. Rupture is sudden, usually associated with hemorrhage and often with extensive laceration beyond the scar.

13.024 Leopold maneuvers allow you to assess:
- A. AP pelvic diameter
- B. lateral pelvic diameter
- C. fetal presentation
- D. quantity of amniotic fluid
- E. frequency and duration of contractions

C is correct.
The four maneuvers allow the examiner to determine presentation, position, and engagement by abdominal exam.

13.025 The MOST common presentation is:
- A. face
- B. limb
- C. transverse
- D. breech
- E. vertex

E is correct.
The vast majority of births are uncomplicated vertex presentations.

TEST PLAN FOR SECTION 13: PREGNANCY, CHILDBIRTH, AND NEONATES

Tasks/areas assessed	Hx and PE	Dx studies	Diagnosis	Prognosis	Management			Applying scientific concepts
					Health maintenance	Clinical intervention	Clinical therapeutics	
Total questions = 25	6	1	1	2	2	2	2	9
Diseases/disorders					*question numbers*			
Adolescent pregnancy								12
Abruptio placentae								22
CNS malformation in fetus								21
Ectopic pregnancy	3							
Incompetent cervix								
Induced abortion								
Infection of the GU tract								
Multiple fetuses								
Placenta previa	4							6
Preeclampsia			11					
Rh incompatibility								
Septic abortion								
Spontaneous abortion	2							
Trisomy								
Unspecified antepartum hemorrhage								23
Other infections complicating pregnancy								
Normal labor and delivery	8,24			19		25		5,9,20
Routine prenatal care	7	1		16	13,14	17	15,18	10

SECTION 14: BLOOD AND BLOOD-FORMING ORGANS

14.001 Which of the following tests would NOT be included in a routine CBC?
  A. total leukocyte count
  B. total erythrocyte count
  C. erythrocyte sedimentation rate
  D. total lymphocyte count
  E. erythrocyte count

C is correct.
The ESR is ordered individually as a nonspecific indication of inflammation.

Use the following information to answer questions 14.002–14.004.

The normal adult values for hemogram and platelet are as follows:			
Test	Female	Male	Units
WBC	4.1–9.3	4.0–9.0	thousand/mm^3
RBC	4.0–5.1	4.5–5.7	million/mm^3
Hgb	12.1–14.9	13.6–16.7	gm/dL
HCT	37–44	40–49	%
MCV	82.2–94.5	82.3–93.2	μm^3
MCH	27.5–32.2	27.8–31.9	pg/cell
MCHC	32.5–35.1	32.8–35.5	gm/dL
Platelet count	130–350	130–350	thousand/mm^3

14.002 A 78-year-old woman was admitted to the hospital from a nursing home for a complete evaluation. She had not been eating properly for several weeks. CBC on admission shows: WBC 12.70, RBC 4.15, Hgb 14.3, HCT 38.9, MCV 70, MCH 32, MCHC 33, platelet count 280,000. Differential: 85% segs, 6% bands, 8% lymphs, 1% monos. This patient has:
  A. leukopenia
  B. neutropenia
  C. leukocytosis and a shift to the left
  D. anemia
  E. thrombocytosis

C is correct.
The WBC is elevated with excess "polys," immature forms, and decreased lymphs. This is termed a "left shift."

14.003 A WBC of 15,500 where there are 15% segs and 85% lymphocytes indicates that the patient has:
  A. leukopenia
  B. immature WBCs
  C. left shift
  D. lymphocytosis

D is correct.
Both the absolute and relative lymphocyte count is increased.

14.004 A patient with a WBC of 13,500 and a differential count of 65% segs, 5% monocytes, and 30% lymphocytes has:
   A. balanced leukopenia
   B. left shift
   C. neutropenia
   D. relative lymphocytosis
   E. balanced leukocytosis

E is correct.
The absolute number of WBCs is abnormally increased, but the differential is normal.

14.005 Epstein-Barr viral infections are associated with increased:
   A. eosinophils
   B. immature neutrophils
   C. lymphocytes
   D. erythrocytes
   E. atypical lymphocytes

E is correct.
Atypical lymphocytes are one of three lab criteria for the diagnosis of mononucleosis.

14.006 Asthma, hay fever, and parasitic infections are associated with:
   A. eosinophilia
   B. neutrophilia
   C. basophilia
   D. atypical lymphocytes
   E. monocytes

A is correct.
Allergy-mediated responses result in increased circulating eosinophils.

14.007 The presence of hypersegmented neutrophils in the peripheral smear may suggest _____ deficiency.
   A. B_{12}
   B. iron
   C. G6PD
   D. hemoglobin

A is correct.
These have four or more lobes in the nucleus.

14.008 The MOST appropriate test for monitoring coumarin therapy is:
   A. APTT
   B. PT
   C. bleeding time
   D. platelet count

B is correct.
Coumarin monitoring with PT is being supplanted by use of the INR, which accounts for variations in the reagents used to conduct the testing.

14.009 Which of the following patient groups should all be screened for anemia (even if asymptomatic)?
   A. school-age children
   B. adults over 40
   C. menstruating females
   D. pregnant females
   E. men over 60

D is correct.
Since there is no clear relationship between symptoms and mild to moderate anemia, routine screening of asymptomatic, nonpregnant patients is not recommended. Iron deficiency anemia is common and amenable to treatment in pregnant women; therefore, screening is recommended.

14.010 Which of the following all produce microcytic anemia?
   A. iron deficiency, anemia of chronic disease, and thalassemia trait
   B. B_{12} deficiency, iron deficiency, and thalassemia trait
   C. folate deficiency, anemia of chronic disease, and liver disease
   D. B_{12} deficiency, liver disease, and anemia of chronic disease
   E. iron deficiency, anemia of chronic disease, and liver disease

A is correct.
Iron deficiency, anemia of chronic disease, and thalassemia trait all produce microcytic anemia. B_{12} deficiency, folate deficiency, and liver disease result in macrocytic anemia.

14.011 The lab test of choice for the diagnosis of iron deficiency anemia is:
   A. hemoglobin
   B. hematocrit
   C. serum ferritin
   D. serum iron
   E. bone marrow aspiration

C is correct.
Ferritin is the storage protein for iron. Its serum level correlates best with marrow stores of iron. It is both sensitive and specific for the diagnosis.

14.012 A 70 year-old woman presents to the ER, complaining of marked fatigue without other symptoms of heart failure. She has a history of chronic stable angina for which she uses sublingual nitro PRN. Vital signs are stable. Other than pale conjunctiva, the physical exam is unremarkable, and her work-up in the ER includes negative CXR, ECG, cardiac enzymes, SMAC, ESR. In the CBC, the only significant findings are Hgb=8 (norm,12–16); HCT=22 (norm, 37–47); MCV=70 (norm, 80–100). You would:
   A. prescribe iron supplements and have patient follow-up with her primary provider in 1 month
   B. prescribe B_{12} and iron and have her follow-up in 1 month
   C. prescribe B_{12} and have her follow-up in 2 weeks
   D. order serum ferritin level and have her follow-up with her primary provider for the results
   E. contact her primary provider to admit her to the hospital for evaluation and treatment

E is correct.
The lab findings suggest iron deficiency anemia. This is best confirmed with a serum ferritin level before treatment is instituted if the patient is stable. In this case, however, the underlying history of cardiac disease and compromised oxygen-carrying capacity (HCT <30) mandate admission for evaluation and consideration of transfusion therapy.

14.013 In a patient presenting with normochromic-normocytic anemia, the NEXT test that classifies these anemias according to the marrow response is the:
   A. ferritin level
   B. reticulocyte count
   C. red cell distribution width (RDW)
   D. Coomb's test
   E. hemoglobin electrophoresis

B is correct.
Reticulocyte counts will classify normochromic-normocytic anemia into two subgroups. If this count is appropriately elevated, the anemia represents hemorrhage or hemolysis. If not, then some type of marrow suppression is the etiology of the anemia.

14.014 Which of the following is FALSE regarding symptoms in patients with anemia?
   A. symptoms are more likely to occur if the onset is precipitous
   B. symptoms of fatigue can be safely attributed to mild iron deficiency anemia in young women
   C. significant anemia may exist without symptoms if the onset is gradual
   D. symptoms in elderly patients require more aggressive investigation and management

B is correct.
A common error among patients is to blame mild anemia for symptoms such as fatigue. This is more likely to represent depression or some other problem and should be carefully investigated.

14.015 The three major criteria for the diagnosis of polycythemia vera are:
   A. leukocytosis, normal SaO$_2$, and hematuria
   B. elevated total red cell volume, normal SaO$_2$, and hematuria
   C. elevated total red cell volume, normal SaO$_2$, and splenomegaly
   D. elevated total white cells, decreased SaO$_2$, and splenomegaly

C is correct.
Elevated total red cell volume, normal SaO$_2$, and splenomegaly are the diagnostic criteria for polycythemia vera. Leukocytosis often does, but need not, occur in association with it. Decreased SaO$_2$ suggests secondary polycythemia. Hematuria suggests a renal etiology, such as renal cell carcinoma, and is not associated with polycythemia vera.

14.016 The primary treatment for polycythemia vera is:
   A. transfusion
   B. volume expansion with crystalloids (normal saline)
   C. phlebotomy
   D. antihistamines

C is correct.
Phlebotomy is the primary mode of therapy. Volume expansion may be used in conjunction, and antihistamines are valuable for controlling associated symptoms of pruritus. Transfusion would be counterproductive in this patient.

14.017 A previously well 4-year-old presents with fever, bleeding, bone pain, generalized lymphadenopathy, splenomegaly, and hepatomegaly. His CBC shows anemia, leukocytosis >100,000, numerous immature WBCs, and thrombocytopenia. The hematologist suggests the prognosis is good. He MOST likely has:
   A. chronic lymphocytic leukemia
   B. acute lymphocytic leukemia
   C. chronic myelocytic (nonlymphocytic) leukemia
   D. acute myelocytic (nonlymphocytic) leukemia

B is correct.
The acute onset, age, and CBC findings suggest ALL in this patient. CLL is typically indolent and affects adults over 50. CML peaks in the 5th decade, is gradual in onset, and often has an associated thrombocytosis. AML primarily affect adults and has a poor prognosis compared with ALL.

14.018 In the lab evaluation of bleeding, the PT assesses the ____, and the PTT assesses the ____.
   A. platelets, intrinsic pathway
   B. extrinsic pathway, platelets
   C. intrinsic pathway, extrinsic pathway
   D. extrinsic pathway, intrinsic pathway

D is correct.   _ Coumadin
The PT assessed the extrinsic clotting pathway, and the PTT the intrinsic pathway. Platelets are better assessed quantitatively via the platelet count and qualitatively by platelet aggregation tests and bleeding time.

14.019 Which is the MOST common type of anemia in women of childbearing age, particularly those who are pregnant?
   A. iron deficiency anemia
   B. thalassemia
   C. sickle cell anemia
   D. pernicious anemia
   E. anemia secondary to folate deficiency

A is correct.
Women of childbearing age have an increased need for iron due to menstrual losses. This is further aggravated by the increased volume of blood needed during pregnancy.

14.020 Management of a patient with sickle cell trait (AS):
- A. is identical with sickle cell disease (SS)
- B. involves only monitoring for infections, as in SS
- C. involves only occasional painful crises compared with SS
- D. is primarily concerned with genetic counseling
- E. dictates avoiding competitive athletics

D is correct.
Sickle trait is an asymptomatic carrier state requiring genetic counseling.

14.021 Which of the following is a cause of microcytic anemia?
- A. B_{12} deficiency
- B. iron deficiency
- C. acute hemorrhage
- D. cirrhosis
- E. aplastic

B is correct.
The others all cause macrocytic.

14.022 Which of the following is a normochromic-normocytic anemia?
- A. chronic disease
- B. folate deficiency
- C. aplastic
- D. sideroblastic
- E. thalassemia trait

A is correct.
Anemia of chronic illness may also be microcytic.

14.023 Which of the following is NOT suggestive of secondary polycythemia?
- A. high-altitude residence
- B. heavy smoker
- C. tollbooth collector
- D. history of murmur
- E. persistent diarrhea

E is correct.
A–D all suggest mechanisms of relative hypoxemia.

14.024 Which statement is FALSE?
- A. anemia is a common condition
- B. there is a clear relationship between mild to moderate anemia and significant symptoms
- C. no clearly measurable benefits from the treatment of mild anemia have been demonstrated
- D. routine screening for anemia in nonpregnant, asymptomatic patients is not recommended
- E. anemia may be secondary to serious underlying disease

B is correct.
Mild or even moderate anemia should not be used to explain symptoms such as fatigue.

14.025 The MOST common initial presentation of sickle cell disease is:
- A. failure to thrive in a child at risk
- B. heavy periods in an adolescent
- C. sudden death in an athlete
- D. painful crisis in an adult
- E. prenatal chorionic biopsy

A is correct.
Sickle cell disease will impact on a child at a young age, with FTT being the most common presentation.

14.026 The test of choice for screening and diagnosis of iron deficiency is:
- A. serum iron
- B. TIBBC
- C. serum ferritin
- D. peripheral smear
- E. folate

C is correct.
Both sensitive and specific for iron deficiency but may be elevated by inflammatory disease or with hepatocellular dysfunction.

14.027 In distinguishing megaloblastic from nonmegaloblastic macrocytic anemia the single MOST helpful test is the:
- A. B_{12} level
- B. folate level
- C. serum ferritin
- D. peripheral smear
- E. hemoglobin electrophoresis

D is correct.
Hypersegmented PMNs are among the earliest and most specific signs of a megaloblastic anemia.

14.028 Groups of drugs that may cause bleeding problems include:
- A. tetracycline, semisynthetic penicillins, cephalosporins
- B. nonsteroidal anti-inflammatories, penicillin VK/G, cephalosporins
- C. nonsteroidal anti-inflammatories, semisynthetic penicillins, sulfas
- D. nonsteroidal anti-inflammatories, semisynthetic penicillins, cephalosporins
- E. nonsteroidal anti-inflammatories, semisynthetic penicillins, diuretics

D is correct.

14.029 A mild anemia with a peripheral smear that shows macrocytosis should make you question the patient carefully about:
- A. smoking
- B. excess carrot consumption
- C. heroin use
- D. alcohol intake
- E. aspirin

D is correct.
Alcohol consumption may result in macrocytic anemia by at least three different mechanisms: folate deficiency, hemorrhage, and chronic liver disease.

14.030 Which of the following would be expected to exhibit symptoms of hemoglobinopathy?
- A. heterozygous sickle (AS)
- B. heterozygous thalassemia (A β-thalassemia)
- C. homozygous (AA)
- D. homozygous sickle (SS)

D is correct.
The homozygous sickle cell patient (SS) has sickle cell disease.

TEST PLAN FOR SECTION 14: BLOOD AND BLOOD-FORMING ORGANS

Tasks/areas assessed	Hx and PE	Dx studies	Diagnosis	Prognosis	Management			Applying scientific concepts
					Health maintenance	Clinical intervention	Clinical therapeutics	
Total questions = 30	5	5	4	0	3	3	2	8
					question numbers			
Diseases/disorders								
Leukemias		1	6,17					2–4
Lymphomas/Hodgkin's		6						
Anemias	14,24,25,29	11,27	7		9,19,26	12,20		10,13,21,22,30
Polycythemia	23	18	15			16		
Coagulation disorder							8,28	
Splenic disorders								
Transfusion reaction								

SECTION 15: INFECTIOUS DISEASES

15.001 Patients being treated with isoniazid (INH) must be advised to avoid:
- A. aspirin
- B. acetaminophen
- C. vitamin B$_6$
- D. rifampin
- E. ibuprofen

B is correct.
Both drugs can be hepatotoxic.

15.002 A 24-year-old man is traveling to a malaria-endemic area. You prescribe antimalarial antibiotics as recommended by the CDC. This represents ____ administration of antibiotics.
- A. therapeutic
- B. empiric
- C. prophylactic

C is correct.
Empiric would be for established infection—organism unknown; therapeutic for established infection—organism known.

15.003 A healthy 18-year-old woman presents, complaining of 1 day of sore throat, runny nose, and fever. She works in a daycare center where several children have been out with streptococcal pharyngitis. She is very anxious that she may have strep and may give it to her boyfriend, who is a PA student and cannot afford to be ill. She also states she cannot afford to be out of work. Which of the following is the MOST important consideration supporting a decision to treat this patient empirically?
- A. anxiety
- B. fever
- C. sore throat
- D. history of exposure
- E. employment

D is correct.
History of strep exposure increases the likelihood of her having strep to the point that empiric therapy is justified.

15.004 The BEST antibiotic listed for chronic bacterial prostatitis is:
- A. amoxicillin-clavulanate (Augmentin®)
- B. trimethoprim/sulfamethoxazole
- C. ceftriaxone (Rocephin®)
- D. azithromycin (Zithromax®)
- E. ciprofloxacin (Cipro®)

E is correct.
It covers the right "bugs" and also penetrates to prostate tissue—a tough job!

15.005 Which type of infection is treated with amphotericin B and fluconazole?
- A. viral
- B. fungal
- C. bacterial
- D. protozoal

B is correct.
These are antifungal agents.

15.006 True statements about AIDS include all of the
following EXCEPT:
- A. the causative agent has been identified as a
  retrovirus
- B. inhalation of virus particles is an important means
  of disease transmission
- C. *Pneumocystis carinii* pneumonia is the most
  common life-threatening opportunistic infection
  complicating AIDS
- D. risk behaviors include anal intercourse and shared
  needles.

B is correct.
Airborne transmission of HIV does not occur.

15.007 Which of the following has NOT been associated
with HIV-impaired immunity?
- A. streptococcal pharyngitis
- B. herpes zoster
- C. genital herpes
- D. tuberculosis

A is correct.
Since we don't develop immunity to group A
strep anyway.

15.008 Treatment for viral pharyngitis may include any
of the following EXCEPT:
- A. penicillin 250 mg QID × 10 days
- B. saline gargles
- C. rest
- D. acetaminophen
- E. fluids

A is correct.
There is no indication for penicillin in viral
pharyngitis.

15.009 There has been an outbreak of a diarrheal illness
in a town in the Adirondacks. Infected persons report
greater than 10 days of diarrhea with associated weight
loss. A common drinking water source is the only factor
shared by all cases. Based on this information, the
etiologic agent is:
- A. *Escherichia coli*
- B. *Clostridium*
- C. *Bacillus cereus*
- D. *Giardia lamblia*

D is correct.
The transmission, location, and clinical
presentation are all consistent with "beaver
fever."

15.010 Which of the following is NOT vaccine
preventable?
- A. rubeola
- B. rubella
- C. parotitis
- D. varicella
- E. mononucleosis

E is correct.
No vaccine is available against Epstein-Barr
virus.

15.011 Koplik's spots are diagnostic for:
- A. rubeola
- B. rubella
- C. parotitis
- D. varicella
- E. mononucleosis

A is correct.
On the buccal mucosa, adjacent to the last
molars. (Not seen very often anymore.)

15.012 The complex of cough, coryza, and conjunctivitis in a patient with fever and a rash is MOST likely:
- A. rubella
- B. rubeola
- C. parotitis
- D. varicella
- E. fifth disease

B is correct.
Accompanied by Koplik's spots to complete the four "C's" (more or less).

15.013 An 11-year-old girl presents with malaise, fever, lymphadenopathy and a diffuse truncal rash. The rash consists of multiple vesicles on an erythematous base. This is MOST likely:
- A. rubella
- B. rubeola
- C. varicella
- D. herpes
- E. zoster

C is correct.
Sometimes called "dewdrops on a rose petal," the rash is diagnostic.

15.014 Which of the following is an appropriate control measure for rubella?
- A. quarantine
- B. passive immunization with immune serum globulin
- C. report to local health department
- D. semiprivate room
- E. exclude all males due to risk of orchitis

C is correct.
Rubella is a reportable disease. Pregnant women and those without adequate immunization should be kept away from the patient. A private room is recommended if the patient is hospitalized, but quarantine is not recommended. Passive immunization of contacts is not generally done. Orchitis is associated with mumps.

15.015 Which immunization would NOT be given to a 20-year-old with no prior history of immunizations?
- A. tetanus
- B. diphtheria
- C. measles
- D. rubella
- E. polio

E is correct.
According to the CDC's ACIP, polio immunizations are not recommended for adults.

15.016 Which of the following would be used to routinely update an adult's tetanus status?
- A. TD
- B. DPT
- C. TIG
- D. Td

D is correct.
TD and DPT contain the higher pediatric doses, and TIG is not routinely used, though it may be indicated in some circumstances.

15.017 Which adult immunization is specifically NOT to be given in the gluteus?
- A. Td
- B. DPT
- C. MMR
- D. hepatitis B

D is correct.
Absorption problems have led to poor antibody response when hepatitis B immunizations are given in the gluteus.

15.018 Unimmunized adults require a primary series of:
- A. two DPTs and a Td
- B. two DPTs and a TD
- C. three DPTs
- D. three TDs
- E. three Tds

E is correct.
The TT (tetanus only) and Td are the only forms used in adults. Primary immunization for both is recommended.

15.019 Causes of false-negative PPDs include all of the following EXCEPT:
   A. immunosuppression
   B. alcoholism
   C. age >45 years
   D. sarcoidosis
   E. BCG vaccination

E is correct.
BCG is an antituberculous vaccine used in some places and results in a false-positive PPD.

15.020 Musculoskeletal manifestations of Lyme disease generally appear in which stage?
   A. early localized infection
   B. early disseminated infection
   C. late localized infection
   D. late persistent infection

D is correct.
Arthralgias, myalgias, and arthritis are common in Lyme.

15.021 The rash of Lyme disease generally appears in which stage?
   A. early localized infection
   B. early disseminated infection
   C. late localized infection
   D. late persistent infection

A is correct.
The erythema chronicum migrans rash (ECM) is usually the presenting complaint in early Lyme. However, not all patients will have the rash.

15.022 Cardiac manifestations of Lyme disease usually present with:
   A. aortic dissection
   B. torsade des pointes
   C. AV block
   D. vegetations on valves
   E. coronary artery aneurysm

C is correct.
In disseminated Lyme, cardiac changes include varying degrees of heart block.

15.023 Which organism is responsible for >50% of all cases of "traveler's diarrhea"?
   A. *E. coli*
   B. *Vibrio cholerae*
   C. *G. lamblia*
   D. *Salmonella*
   E. *Campylobacter jejuni*

A is correct.
E. coli diarrhea is the most common and has all sorts of great names like "Montezuma's revenge."

15.024 Which of the following is likely to turn stools black?
   A. diphenoxylate (Lomotil®)
   B. bismuth subsalicylate (Pepto-Bismol®)
   C. kaolin/pectin (Kaopectate®)
   D. loperamide (Imodium®)
   E. Pedialyte®

B is correct.
Remember to warn patients if they haven't used this before, because you're probably telling them to watch for signs of blood (like melena).

15.025 Which of the following is the hemorrhagic fever virus associated with ARDS?
   A. dengue
   B. Hanta
   C. Lassa
   D. Marburg
   E. Ebola

B is correct.
Outbreaks in the Southwest U.S. have made us more aware of the Hantavirus. Of all of these, I've only seen one case (dengue), but the others make good books and movies.

15.026 Which of the following bites is considered as high risk for transmitting rabies?
A. skunk
B. squirrel
C. rat
D. spider
E. human

A is correct.
Also bats, foxes, and a particular problem for us in New York, raccoons.

15.027 Patients with mononucleosis and grossly enlarged tonsils are best treated with:
A. acyclovir (Zovirax®)
B. amoxicillin
C. immunoglobulin
D. NSAIDs
E. steroids

E is correct.
With airway compromise as the primary concern, steroids are rapidly effective in reducing tonsillar inflammation.

15.028 The BEST antibiotic listed for the treatment of early Lyme disease in an adult is:
A. penicillin
B. trimethoprim/sulfamethoxazole
C. erythromycin
D. doxycycline
E. nitrofurantoin

D is correct.
The others are not effective against the spirochete, although historically penicillin seemed to work in children for a while in the early New Jersey outbreaks.

15.029 AIDS is
A. a virus
B. a bacteria
C. a disease
D. a syndrome
E. none of the above

D is correct.
AIDS is the syndrome; HIV is the virus. (Need an easy one occasionally)

15.030 In the lab evaluation of an HIV patient, ____ count <200 or 14% is a diagnostic marker for AIDS.
A. CD4
B. total lymphocytes
C. WBC
D. RBC
E. ELISA

A is correct.
This type of lymphocyte is specifically followed to monitor the progression of the disease.

15.031 "P24" measures:
A. antibodies
B. lymphocytes
C. T cells
D. T-helper cells
E. viral particles

E is correct.
A direct measure of antigen, it quantifies viral load.

15.032 HIV primarily affects which type of immunity?
A. humoral
B. cellular

B is correct.
Thus, the marker diseases are those against which the body is protected by lymphocytes.

15.033 When doing a PPD on an HIV-infected patient:
A. use two controls (usually *Candida* and mumps)
B. use a *Candida* control
C. use a mumps control
D. use no control

A is correct.
Controls are necessary to avoid false-negatives due to immune suppression.

15.034 Your patient reports his confidential HIV test done in Albany was negative. Which of the following interpretations is NOT possible?
    A. the patient is not infected
    B. the patient was infected within 4–6 weeks of testing
    C. the patient may be infected but have a false-negative test
    D. the patient may have advanced disease
    E. all of the above are possible interpretations

E is correct.
All of these scenarios are possible in the patient with a single negative test.

15.035 Which of the following is MOST frequently associated with folliculitis?
    A. *Staphylococcus aureus*
    B. *Pseudomonas aeruginosa*
    C. *Candida albicans*
    D. *E. coli*

A is correct.
Less common "hot-tub folliculitis" is caused by *Pseudomonas*.

15.036 Which of the following statements is TRUE about infectious mononucleosis?
    A. it is caused by cytomegalovirus
    B. it is diagnosed most commonly in preschoolers
    C. SMAC may have elevated LFTs
    D. CBC will have an elevated number of monocytes

C is correct.
Mono will commonly cause liver inflammation leading to elevated LFTs.

15.037 Important aspects to consider when providing pretest counseling to a possible HIV/AIDS patient include:
    A. confidentiality
    B. stress related to a positive test result
    C. risk behaviors
    D. all of the above

D is correct.
New York state and other agencies provide specific training for HIV testing. I highly recommend it.

15.038 Fluids considered to be at risk for transmission of HIV are:
    A. tears, synovial fluid, vaginal secretions, semen, blood
    B. CSF, urine, vaginal secretions, semen, blood
    C. CSF, synovial fluid, stool, semen, blood
    D. CSF, synovial fluid, vaginal secretions, saliva, blood
    E. CSF, synovial fluid, vaginal secretions, semen, blood

E is correct.
See question 15.039.

15.039 Fluids NOT considered at risk for HIV transmission, unless containing visible amounts of blood:
    A. tears, saliva, urine, stool
    B. amniotic fluid, saliva, urine, stool
    C. tears, CSF, urine, stool
    D. tears, saliva, vaginal secretions, stool
    E. tears, saliva, urine, synovial fluid

A is correct.
Any questions?

15.040 The first test usually performed for screening HIV is:
   A. Western blot
   B. HIV antigen
   C. ELISA or EIA
   D. PCR
   E. none of the above

C is correct.
The ELISA test is more sensitive, though less specific, than the confirmatory test.

15.041 The confirmatory test after two positive screening tests is:
   A. ELISA
   B. PCR
   C. Western blot
   D. EIA
   E. none of the above

C is correct.
The Western blot is highly specific and rules out false-positives from the highly sensitive ELISA.

15.042 ELISA antibody testing assesses:
   A. IgE
   B. IgG
   C. IgM
   D. IgA

B is correct.
Thus, the "window period" of false-negative tests between infection and development of sufficient antibody to convert the test to positive.

15.043 Initial lab assessment of a HIV positive patient includes:
   A. Hx, PE, pelvic, PAP, CXR
   B. STD screening
   C. CBC and diff, CD4, CD8, T cell, Hep B&C, PPD, and anergy panel
   D. toxoplasmosis, CMV
   E. all of the above

E is correct.
A thorough baseline needs to be established and subclinical disease to be treated before the immune system becomes impaired.

15.044 PAP smears in women who are HIV positive should be done:
   A. monthly
   B. q6–12 months
   C. annually
   D. annually for 3 years, then biannually if negative
   E. biannually

B is correct.
More frequent monitoring is required.

15.045 A 15-year-old boy develops fever and tachypnea following 5 days of sore throat, headache, and gradually worsening cough. The CXR shows bilateral infiltrates. WBC is normal. The MOST likely diagnosis is:
   A. pneumococcal pneumonia
   B. mycoplasmal pneumonia
   C. tuberculosis
   D. gram-negative pneumonia

B is correct.
Mycoplasmal pneumonia is the most common pneumonia in this age group, and consistent with the work-up.

15.046 The BEST drug listed for treating the patient in 15.045 would be:
   A. penicillin
   B. erythromycin
   C. TMP/SMX
   D. cefaclor (Ceclor®)

B is correct.
Erythromycin and the other macrolides provide the best efficacy against *Mycoplasma*.

15.047 Besides myalgias, nausea, and vomiting, AZT (zidovudine/Retrovir®) side effects are primarily:
    A. neurological
    B. hematological
    C. ototoxic
    D. renal
    E. dermatological

B is correct.
AZT is associated with hematological toxicity, including granulocytopenia and severe anemia.

15.048 AZT is used to treat HIV infections because it:
    A. prevents HIV from entering lymphocytes by altering the permeability of the cell membranes
    B. has been shown to prolong life, although its precise action is not known
    C. inhibits reverse transcriptase and alters viral DNA so that it cannot replicate
    D. is viricidal

C is correct.
Kind of like inserting the wrong ledders in werds.

15.049 Chronic suppressive acyclovir (Zovirax®) therapy is appropriate for:
    A. all patients with genital herpes
    B. an individual who wants to prevent a genital herpes outbreak during a vacation
    C. a person whose recurrences are marked by pain, fever, or systemic symptoms
    D. a pregnant woman, to prevent an outbreak close to the time of delivery

C is correct.
Pregnancy category C. Let the OB decide.

15.050 A 59-year-old man with severe alcoholism presents, complaining of cough for 10 days. He is now short of breath and feverish and has pleuritic pain with the cough. He has been coughing up dark reddish-brown sputum for 2 days. He is ill-appearing and febrile (101°F). On a sputum Gram stain, you find many gram-negative rods. His CXR shows consolidation in the RML with a possible area of cavitation. Which type of pneumonia does this MOST likely represent?
    A. viral
    B. *Klebsiella pneumoniae*
    C. *Streptococcus pneumoniae*
    D. *Mycoplasma pneumoniae*
    E. *Legionella pneumophila*

B is correct.
The alcoholic history and the CXR appearance suggest the diagnosis. The sputum rules out strep, *Mycoplasma*, and *Legionella*, if the organism seen is the etiologic agent.

15.051 CXR findings are disproportionately MORE severe than the clinical picture in which type of pneumonia?
    A. *Haemophilus influenzae*
    B. aspiration
    C. pneumococcal
    D. mycoplasmal

D is correct.
Diffuse, patchy infiltrates on the CXR correlate poorly with clinically less severe disease, hence the old name "walking pneumonia."

15.052 In HIV patients Bactrim® prophylaxis is used for:
A. PCP
B. toxoplasmosis
C. CMV infection
D. A and B
E. all of the above

D is correct.
Trimethoprim/sulfamethoxazole to the more formal provider.

15.053 Adverse reactions to trimethoprim/sulfamethoxazole in HIV-positive patients are:
A. increased in incidence
B. potentially severe, including Steven-Johnson syndrome
C. commonly rashes
D. A and C
E. all of the above

E is correct.
Also Septra®. (But you knew that.)

15.054 In a 8-year-old patient who is allergic to penicillin, which of the following drugs would you utilize to treat a streptococcal pharyngitis?
A. tetracycline
B. erythromycin
C. a third-generation cephalosporin
D. gentamicin

B is correct.
AHA recommends erythromycin as the treatment of choice for penicillin-allergic patients.

15.055 Antihistamines that may produce life-threatening arrhythmias when combined with systemic antifungals and erythromycin include:
A. clemastine (Tavist®)
B. astemizole (Hismanal®)
C. diphenhydramine (Benadryl®)
D. A and B
E. all of the above

B is correct.
Torsade des pointes is the primary, but not only, dysrhythmia noted.

15.056 Acute HIV infection is MOST similar to:
A. mononucleosis
B. strep pharyngitis
C. chicken pox
D. flu
E. measles

A is correct.
Makes for a scary differential in young, sexually active adults.

15.057 Lab findings helpful in distinguishing HIV from EBV include:
A. differential WBC count, heterophile titer
B. total WBCs, lymphocytes
C. thrombocytes, lymphocytes
D. total WBCs, heterophile titer
E. differential WBC count, total WBCs

A is correct.
HIV will not result in the "typical" atypical lymphocytes of IM, nor will it elevate the heterophile antibody titer.

15.058 Oral findings that suggest a patient has EBV rather than acute HIV are:
A. exudative tonsils and oral ulcers
B. nonexudative tonsils and no oral ulcers
C. nonexudative tonsils and oral ulcers
D. exudative tonsils and no oral ulcers

D is correct.
A patient with EBV is more likely to have exudative tonsils and no oral ulcers. With HIV, nonexudative tonsils with oral ulcers is more common.

15.059 The MOST common CXR finding in a patient with PCP is:
   A. normal
   B. RML infiltrate
   C. lingular pneumonia
   D. unilateral upper infiltrates

A is correct.
Remember CXR findings commonly lag behind the clinical disease. If it is apparent, changes are usually diffuse, interstitial, and bilateral.

15.060 Primary symptom in esophageal candidiasis is:
   A. dysphagia
   B. reflux
   C. odynophagia
   D. regurgitation
   E. vomiting

C is correct.
Pain on swallowing in an HIV patient should prompt a search for esophageal candidiasis, a common part of AIDS.

15.061 Aphthous ulcers in an AIDS patient may be managed with:
   A. topical anesthetics
   B. topical steroids
   C. systemic steroids
   D. A and B
   E. all of the above

E is correct.
Aggressive therapy may be required, as lesions can be so severe as to impair adequate oral intake.

TEST PLAN FOR SECTION 15: INFECTIOUS DISEASES

Tasks/areas assessed	Hx and PE	Dx studies	Diagnosis	Prognosis	Management Health maintenance	Clinical intervention	Clinical therapeutics	Applying scientific concepts
Total questions = 61	2	9	10	2	12	3	11	12
Diseases/disorders					*question numbers*			
STDs								
AIDS		30,31,40,41	43,55	34	7,37,39,44,51,53	48	46,52,54,60	6,29,32,33,38,42,47
Infectious mononucleosis	57	36,56			10		27	
Lyme disease		22					28	20,21
Mumps								
Rabies				26				
Rubella						14		
Rubeola	11		12					
Varicella			13					
Other viral diseases/*Chlamydia*		58	25,45		15–18,49		8,61	
Other IDs		59	9,23,35,50			3	1,2,4	5,19,24

SECTION 16: INJURIES, WOUNDS, TOXIC EFFECTS, AND BURNS

16.001 First antibiotic of choice for dental problems is:
A. penicillin
B. tetracycline
C. erythromycin
D. sulfa

A is correct.
Pen VK provides good coverage for oral infections in immunocompetent hosts.

16.002 ER management of acute tooth pain includes:
A. extractions
B. debridement
C. nerve blocks
D. antibiotics

D is correct.
Control infection with ABOs and pain with analgesics in the acute setting, and refer to the dentist for definitive care.

16.003 Chronic tooth pain can often be treated with:
A. dental floss
B. brushing
C. antiseptic rinses
D. systemic analgesics

A is correct.
Dental floss may remove accumulated food particles, a source of inflammation, and thereby reduce some chronic pain. Brushing and rinsing may help but may not get to trapped debris. Systemic analgesics should not be used chronically.

16.004 Avulsed permanent teeth should NOT be:
A. cleaned
B. replaced in the socket
C. transported in milk
D. transported in dry gauze

D is correct.
Avulsed teeth should be cleaned and replaced in their socket immediately if possible. If not, they may be transported in a container of milk. (Skim if the patient is dieting.)

16.005 A 3-year-old child fell backward from a seated position, striking his head on the linoleum floor. He cried immediately and did not at any time lose consciousness. There is a 3-cm "lump" in the occipital scalp without lacerations or deformities. His neurological exam is normal. He is not taking any medications. Which of the following is indicated?
A. skull tomograms
B. plain skull films
C. CT scan
D. MRI scan
E. none of the above

E is correct.
A negative neurological exam without loss of consciousness means radiological studies are not indicated in this patient.

16.006 The BEST method of treatment for anterior epistaxis is:
A. ice
B. tilting the head back
C. direct pressure on nares
D. Neo-Synephrine®

C is correct.
Direct pressure will control most epistaxis. Ice and Neo-Synephrine® may be helpful as well. Do not tip the head back.

16.007 In a patient with jaw pain, which of the following will suggest TMJ syndrome vs. acute myocardial infarction:
    A. open 1.5 inches without deviation
    B. tenderness of muscles
    C. tingling in fingers
    D. chest tightness
    E. ringing in one ear

B is correct.
Jaw pain in AMI is referred, and therefore the muscles should be nontender. In TMJ syndrome, spasm and tenderness of the masseters is expected.

16.008 Which is TRUE regarding alkali burns to the eye?
    A. they are less serious than acid burns
    B. they should be irrigated with a weak acid
    C. they should be irrigated with a strong acid
    D. they should not be irrigated with a Morgan lens
    E. irrigation should continue until pH is normalized

E is correct.
Acids should not be used to irrigate eyes. Alkali burns can be more serious than some acid burns. A Morgan lens is a useful device for prolonged irrigations, as might be needed here.

16.009 In fluid resuscitation, the major difference between crystalloids and colloids is that:
    A. crystalloids leave the vascular space more readily
    B. colloids leave the vascular space more readily
    C. crystalloids seldom enter the extracellular space
    D. colloids are essentially water and salt
    E. crystalloids contain large protein molecules

A is correct.
Crystalloids, which are composed of water and electrolytes, leave the intravascular compartment rapidly.

16.010 Complications of Ringer's lactate solution may include:
    A. respiratory acidosis
    B. respiratory alkalosis
    C. metabolic alkalosis
    D. metabolic acidosis

C is correct.
Since lactate is metabolized to bicarbonate; large quantities may increase the blood's pH—a metabolic alkalosis.

16.011 BEST use of crystalloids is:
    A. rapid volume expansion up to 2000 cc
    B. volume replacement with clotting disorders
    C. volume expansion up to 12 L
    D. treatment for low hematocrit

A is correct.
Some centers still prefer colloids for volume expansion. The debate goes on...

16.012 Colloids:
    A. produce more peripheral edema
    B. are more complicated if capillary leakage is occurring
    C. diffuse more rapidly into extracellular space
    D. are used for maintenance fluids
    E. none of the above

B is correct.
Because colloids contain osmotically active proteins, if they leak into areas where they aren't wanted (e.g., intra-alveolar), they draw water with them and are more difficult for the body to reabsorb.

16.013 Causes of hypokalemia may include all of the following EXCEPT:
    A. loop diuretics
    B. metabolic acidosis
    C. NG suctioning
    D. inadequate dietary intake
    E. diarrhea

B is correct.
Increased loss (diuresis or diarrhea) or decreased intake (inadequate diet) result in a net loss of potassium. Metabolic acidosis may cause potassium concentrations to shift across compartments with no net gain/loss.

16.014 Foreign bodies of the cornea are BEST seen by:
   A. hand-held ophthalmoscope
   B. fluorescein staining and UV light
   C. x-rays
   D. bright direct light

B is correct.
Fluorescein will cause corneal foreign bodies to stand out under UV light and provide the patient a psychedelic orange stripe into the ipsilateral ear.

16.015 A pedestrian struck by a car has stridorous respirations and a large bleeding laceration on the thigh. Your first priority is to:
   A. control the bleeding
   B. hyperoxygenate
   C. replace fluids
   D. secure the airway

D is correct.
ATLS protocols require that securing an adequate airway is the first priority in a trauma patient. Stridorous respirations suggest partial upper airway obstruction.

16.016 In the assessment of abdominal trauma in the ER, the goal is:
   A. a specific diagnosis
   B. to rule out ruptured spleen
   C. to rule out perforation
   D. to determine whether intra-abdominal injury requiring surgery exists

D is correct.
A specific diagnosis is often not possible, but the need for emergency surgical intervention must be ascertained.

16.017 Aspiration of gross blood during diagnostic peritoneal lavage is:
   A. always clinically significant
   B. diagnostic of ruptured spleen
   C. diagnostic of ruptured hollow viscus
   D. sometimes a false-positive finding

A is correct.
Choices with always or never are never the right answer.

16.018 The BEST way to confirm a tension pneumothorax in the ER is:
   A. the rush of air when you insert a needle
   B. inspiratory/expiratory portable CXRs
   C. PA and lateral CXR in radiology
   D. portable AP CXR

A is correct.
You don't have time for anything else.

16.019 Bowel sounds in the chest of a trauma victim suggest:
   A. intra-abdominal bleeding leading to hyperactivity
   B. ruptured diaphragm
   C. hemothorax
   D. tension pneumothorax

B is correct.
Bowel can herniate into the thorax after diaphragmatic injury, particularly deceleration injury.

16.020 The BEST way to confirm a cardiac tamponade in the ER is:
   A. the rush of blood when you insert a needle
   B. echocardiogram
   C. cardiac monitor
   D. 12-lead ECG
   E. portable AP CXR

A is correct.
You don't have time for anything else.

16.021 Which burns are usually MOST painful?
   A. superficial partial thickness
   B. deep partial thickness
   C. full thickness

A is correct.
Burns become less sensitive as they go deeper and destroy skin pain receptors.

16.022 Lidocaine with epinephrine may be used to suture an actively bleeding _____ injury.
   A. finger
   B. toe
   C. scalp
   D. thumb

C is correct.
Lidocaine with epinephrine should not be used in the extremities, as vascular compromise is possible.

16.023 The initial treatment of tension pneumothorax is needle decompression by insertion into:
   A. the second intercostal space in the midclavicular line
   B. the first intercostal space in the midclavicular line
   C. the second intercostal space in the anterior axillary line
   D. the first intercostal space in the anterior axillary line
   E. the third intercostal space at the sternal border

A is correct.

16.024 An adult patient has a burn on the leg resulting from the spill of a pot of coffee. The wound on the upper and lower right leg is bright red and has various-sized bullae that are moist and weeping. The burns are hypersensitive. This burn could be considered :
   A. superficial partial thickness
   B. deep partial thickness
   C. full thickness
   D. fourth degree

A is correct.
The appearance and sensitivity are the clues.

16.025 In a patient with a deep partial thickness wound, all of the following measures to prevent infection are indicated EXCEPT:
   A. tetanus booster PRN
   B. debridement of blisters
   C. bacteriostatic ointments
   D. dressing changes
   E. oral antibiotics

E is correct.
Prophylactic antibiotics are not indicated.

16.026 Which of the following is NOT suggestive of developing infection in a burn wound?
   A. pain
   B. swelling
   C. itching
   D. erythema
   E. lymphangitis

C is correct.
Significant itching is common during the healing process.

16.027 Using the rule of nines, in a patient who has burns over the entire right and left leg and the anterior chest and abdomen, what percentage of his body surface is burned?
   A. 18%
   B. 25%
   C. 36%
   D. 45%
   E. 54%

E is correct.
18% each for the legs and 18% for the anterior thorax.

16.028 Using the rule of nines, an adult who has burns over the right anterior arm and the right anterior leg would have approximately what percentage of his body burned?
    A. 6%
    B. 13.5%
    C. 18%
    D. 27%

B is correct.
4.5% for half an arm plus 9% for half a leg.

16.029 Which swallowed foreign body is MOST serious?
    A. watch battery
    B. ornamental pearl
    C. coin
    D. marble

A is correct.
Watch batteries may release corrosives that can burn and scar the tissues. They are prone to become lodged at the GE junction and can result in serious complications.

TEST PLAN FOR SECTION 16: INJURIES, WOUND, TOXIC EFFECTS, AND BURNS

Tasks/areas assessed	Hx and PE	Dx studies	Diagnosis	Prognosis	Management			Applying scientific concepts
					Health maintenance	Clinical intervention	Clinical therapeutics	
Total questions = 29	0	2	5	1	1	9	4	7
Diseases/disorders				_question numbers_				
Cranial or ocular injury		5						
Epistaxis						6	9	
Eye burn								
Foreign body in eye/ear/nose		15						
Foreign body in trachea (aspiration)								
Swallowed foreign body								29
Traumatic pneumothorax						19,24		
Various open wounds						23		22,28
Other burns			25	27			26	
Adverse effects of medicines								
Drug overdose								
Toxic effects of other substances								
Postoperative trauma			7,8		3	2,4	1	14
Other/miscellaneous emergency problems						16,17,21		
Other trauma			18,20				10	11-13

SECTION 17: ILL-DEFINED SYMPTOM COMPLEXES

17.001 A 4-year-old white male presents to the ER with stridor for 1 hour. Stridor is MOST suggestive of:
   A. lower respiratory infection
   B. upper respiratory infection
   C. upper airway obstruction
   D. small airways disease
   E. bronchospasm

C is correct.
Stridor is a high-pitched inspiratory sound suggestive of upper airway obstruction. Upper respiratory infection generally does not produce adventitious lung sounds. Lower respiratory infections most often result in rhonchi and/or rales, while small airways disease such as asthma commonly presents with wheezing.

17.002 Approximately what percentage of patients with septic shock will die?
   A. nearly 0%
   B. 25%
   C. 50%
   D. 5%
   E. nearly 100%

C is correct.
Sepsis, even with appropriate care, has a high mortality rate.

17.003 All of the following are appropriate measures to reduce fever in a patient EXCEPT:
   A. acetaminophen
   B. sponge bath with tepid water
   C. sponge bath with alcohol
   D. remove excess clothing and covering from the patient

C is correct.
An old-time remedy, cooling the skin with rubbing alcohol is not significantly better than using water, and it can be absorbed through the skin, causing toxicity.

17.004 Of the following causes of sepsis, which is MOST likely to progress to septic shock?
   A. fungal
   B. viral
   C. parasitic
   D. gram-negative bacterial
   E. gram-positive bacterial

D is correct.
Toxins produced by gram-negative bacteria are responsible for much of the pathophysiology of sepsis.

17.005 Which of the following is NOT one of the diagnostic criteria for sepsis?
   A. identified nidus of infection
   B. temperature >38°C or <36°C
   C. pulse >90 bpm
   D. respirations >20/min or $PaCO_2$ <32
   E. WBCs>12,000 or bands >10%

A is correct.
In many cases, a site of infection can not be identified.

17.006 Which of the following defines the progression from sepsis to severe sepsis?
   A. identified nidus of infection
   B. hypotension
   C. pulse >100 bpm
   D. respirations >24/min or $PaCO_2$ <28
   E. WBCs >20,000 or bands >15%

B is correct.
Hypotension is the key to prognosis and represents vascular collapse, an ominous sign in a septic patient.

17.007 Which of the following is the MOST common cause of septic shock?
- A. trauma
- B. burns
- C. pancreatitis
- D. fungal infection
- E. bacterial infection

E is correct.
Think of gram-negative infections in compromised hosts.

17.008 Which of the following is LEAST likely to be a cardiac complaint?
- A. chest pain
- B. weakness
- C. vertigo
- D. syncope
- E. back pain

C is correct.
True vertigo (as opposed to dizziness) is usually the result of an otological problem.

17.009 Which of the following is required in making the diagnosis of costochondritis?
- A. reproducible chest wall tenderness on palpation
- B. reproducible pain with respiration
- C. reproducible pain with exertion
- D. reproducible pain with movement

A is correct.
Pain with respiration can be musculoskeletal or pleuritic. Pain on exertion suggests angina, and pain on movement is usually musculoskeletal, but not as specific as localized tenderness to palpation.

17.010 Oral hairy leukoplakia (HL):
- A. involves predominantly the lateral tongue
- B. is rare in immunocompetent patients
- C. often requires no therapy
- D. is probably caused by EBV
- E. all of the above

E is correct.
Asymptomatic verrucous, white patches that don't rub off—a common manifestation of HIV disease.

17.011 HL can be BEST be distinguished from oral candidiasis by:
- A. clinical appearance
- B. scraping (HL doesn't come off)
- C. KOH
- D. biopsy

D is correct.
Particularly since the two can occur together and have a similar appearance, biopsy is the surest way.

17.012 The MOST common clinical manifestation of AIDS in the absence of prophylaxis is:
- A. oral candidiasis
- B. lymphadenopathy
- C. Kaposi's sarcoma
- D. oral hairy leukoplakia
- E. PCP

E is correct.
Trimethoprim/sulfamethoxazole prophylaxis is commonly used.

17.013 Kaposi's sarcoma can involve:
- A. head, neck, and trunk
- B. mucous membranes
- C. lymph nodes
- D. GI tract and lung
- E. all of the above

E is correct.
Brown to purple nodules anywhere on the body.

17.014 Abdominal pain from distention of hollow organs is termed:
   A. visceral
   B. parietal
   C. somatic
   D. mechanical
   E. inflammation

A is correct.
Characteristics of abdominal pain are important clues to the diagnosis.

17.015 Pain from inflammation of abdominal organs is termed:
   A. visceral
   B. parietal
   C. somatic
   D. mechanical

C is correct.
Causes of somatic pain can be distinguished from causes of visceral pain.

17.016 Which of the following is a cause of somatic pain?
   A. adhesions
   B. gallstones
   C. appendilith
   D. pancreatitis

D is correct.
A–C initially cause obstruction and therefore distention (visceral pain).

17.017 When the small bowel becomes hyperdynamic, the pain is perceived to be:
   A. epigastric
   B. periumbilical
   C. RUQ
   D. RLQ
   E. LUQ

B is correct.
As in the initial presentation of appendicitis.

17.018 Referred pain is perceived in:
   A. the peritoneum overlying the involved organ
   B. the structures immediately around the inflamed tissue
   C. the area of embryological origin of the organ
   D. none of the above

C is correct.
This accounts for some of the more unusual presentations, such as shoulder pain in ruptured spleen.

17.019 When the gallbladder becomes hyperdynamic, the pain is perceived to be:
   A. epigastric
   B. periumbilical
   C. RUQ
   D. RLQ
   E. LUQ

A is correct.
Precipitated by obstruction, localization follows the development of inflammation.

17.020 When the appendix becomes hyperdynamic, the pain is perceived to be:
   A. epigastric
   B. periumbilical
   C. RUQ
   D. RLQ
   E. LUQ

B is correct.
Most commonly in response to a fecalith.

17.021 Somatic pain is:
  A. transient
  B. poorly localized
  C. perceived in the area of embryological origin
  D. colicky
  E. identified by pointing with one finger to point of maximum intensity

E is correct.
Somatic pain is well localized.

17.022 In general, for hollow organs:
  A. somatic pain represents mechanical events
  B. visceral pain represents inflammation
  C. A and B
  D. somatic pain represents inflammation and visceral pain represents mechanical events

D is correct.
Generally sums it up.

17.023 An 18-year-old woman with a history of recurrent UTIs presents with localized left CVA pain that came on gradually and is dull and achy in nature. She MOST likely has:
  A. cholelithiasis
  B. small bowel obstruction
  C. nephrolithiasis
  D. pyelonephritis

D is correct.
The patient has somatic pain. A–C cause visceral pain.

inflammation

mechanical

17.024 A 27-year-old man presents, complaining of severe, colicky pain in the right flank radiating to the groin. He MOST likely has:
  A. renal colic
  B. pyelonephritis
  C. pancreatitis
  D. cholecystitis

A is correct.
Obstructive symptoms mean visceral pain.

17.025 GERD in small children may present with:
  A. failure to thrive
  B. chronic bronchitis
  C. A or B
  D. none of the above

C is correct.
Bronchial irritation due to aspiration.

17.026 Nonmedical management of reflux disease involves:
  A. weight reduction
  B. avoidance of large meals prior to bedtime
  C. lowering the head of the bed
  D. A and B
  E. all of the above

D is correct.
Raise the head of the bed.

17.027 Other methods of nonmedical management to be initially utilized include avoiding:
  A. cigarettes
  B. alcohol
  C. coffee
  D. A and B
  E. all of the above

D is correct.

17.028 Probably, the MOST important and/or dangerous-to-miss "mimic" of reflux disease to consider in the differential diagnosis is:
- A. peptic ulcer disease
- B. esophageal spasm
- C. myocardial ischemia
- D. cholelithiasis

C is correct.
Patients with inferior wall ischemia may have epigastric symptoms described as "heartburn."

17.029 In suspected GI bleeds, measurement of the hematocrit in the acute phase of blood loss:
- A. is the most accurate means of determining degree of blood loss
- B. may show deceptively little decline
- C. is important as a baseline to establish future loss
- D. B and C

D is correct.
Acute losses may not be reflected by the hematocrit early on.

17.030 Patients require transfusion:
- A. if their hematocrit declines below 30%
- B. if their hematocrit declines 5% within 24 hours
- C. if their hematocrit declines below 28%
- D. only if they are symptomatic or hemodynamically unstable
- E. none of the above

D is correct.
Transfusion is avoided unless absolutely necessary to prevent complications.

TEST PLAN FOR SECTION 17: ILL-DEFINED SYMPTOM COMPLEXES

Tasks/areas assessed	Hx and PE	Dx studies	Diagnosis	Prognosis	Management			Applying scientific concepts
					Health maintenance	Clinical intervention	Clinical therapeutics	
Total questions = 30	6	2	7	2	0	3	1	9
					question numbers			
Diseases/disorders								
Bacterial infections								
Viremia	10							
Anorexia								
Weight fluctuation								
Murmurs								
Palpitations								
Cough			25					
Dyspnea								1,12
Stridor								
Dyspepsia		29	28			26,27	30	
Dysphagia								
GI hemorrhage								
Ascites								
Hepatomegaly								
Dysuria								
Renal colic			24					

(continued on next page)

TEST PLAN FOR SECTION 17 (continued)

Tasks/areas assessed	Hx and PE	Dx studies	Diagnosis	Prognosis	Management			Applying scientific concepts
					Health maintenance	Clinical intervention	Clinical therapeutics	
Abdominal mass								
Abdominal pain	17,19,20		23					14–16,18,21,22
Allergy								
Chest pain	8		9					
Convulsions								
Developmental problems								
Dizziness/giddiness								
Edema								
Enlarged lymph nodes	13	11						
Headache								
Lack of normal physiological development								
Lymphadenitis, except mesenteric								
Malaise and fatigue								
Migraine						3		
Pyrexia, origin unknown								
Reyes syndrome								
Septic shock			5,6	2,4				7
Sleep disturbances								
Syncope and collapse								

BIBLIOGRAPHY

Algranati PS. *The Pediatric Patient: An Approach to History and Physical Examination.* Baltimore: Williams and Wilkins, 1992.

American Heart Association. *Textbook of Advanced Cardiac Life Support.* AHA: Dallas, TX, 1994.

Bates B. *A Guide to Physical Examination and History Taking*, 6th ed. Philadelphia: JB Lippincott, 1995.

Behrman R, Kleigman R, Arvin A, eds. *Nelson Textbook of Pediatrics,* 15th ed. Philadelphia: WB Saunders, 1996.

Chernecky C, Krech R, Berger B. *Laboratory Tests and Diagnostic Procedures.* Philadelphia: WB Saunders, 1993.

Dubin D. *Rapid Interpretation of EKG's*, 4th ed. Tampa, FL: Cover Publishing, 1989.

Ewald G, McKenzie C, eds. *Manual of Medical Therapeutics*, 28th ed. Boston: Little, Brown, 1995.

Goroll AH, May LA, Mulley AG Jr, eds. *Primary Care Medicine, Office Evaluation of the Adult Patient*, 3rd ed. Philadelphia: JB Lippincott, 1995.

Hoppenfeld S. *Physical Examination of the Spine and Extremities.* Norwalk, CT: Appleton & Lange, 1976.

Isselbacher KJ, et al, eds. *Harrison's Principles of Internal Medicine,* 13th ed. New York: McGraw-Hill, 1994.

Kumar V, Cotran R, Robbins S. *Basic Pathology*, 5th. ed. Philadelphia: WB Saunders, 1992.

Leitman M. *Manual for Eye Examination and Diagnosis,* 4th. ed. Williston, VT: Blackwell Scientific Publications, 1994.

Nealon T, Nealon W. *Fundamental Skills in Surgery,* 4th ed. Philadelphia: WB Saunders, 1994.

Noble J, ed. *Textbook of Primary Care Medicine.* St. Louis, MO: Mosby-Yearbook, 1996.

Pernoll M, ed. *Current Obstetric and Gynecologic Diagnosis and Treatment,* 8th ed. Norwalk, CT: Appleton & Lange, 1994.

Way LW. *Current Surgical Diagnosis and Therapy,* 10th ed. Norwalk, CT: Appleton & Lange, 1994.